bird's eye view

Stories of a life
lived in health care.

by Sue Robins

Published in 2019 by Bird Communications.
Vancouver, Canada

First edition.

Publisher's Cataloging-in-Publication Data

Robins, Sue, author.
Bird's eye view : stories of a life lived in health care / Sue Robins.

Robins, Sue–Health–Anecdotes.
Breast–Cancer–Patients–Canada–Anecdotes.
Breast–Cancer–Patients–Canada–Biography.
Children with Down syndrome–Canada–Anecdotes.
Patient-centered health care–Canada–Anecdotes.
Breast cancer patients' writings, Canadian.

ISBN: 978-1-9991560-1-5 (trade paper)
ISBN: 978-1-9991560-2-2 (e-book)

Editorial services from Hambone Publishing, Melbourne, Australia. Illustrations by Jacqueline Robins. Book cover and interior design by Aaron Mumby Design. Photography by Ryan Walter Wagner.

For more information on bulk orders, or to enquire about bringing the author to your event, email book@birdcommunications.ca.

To my Mike.

Table of Contents

And when we speak we are afraid
our words will not be heard
nor welcomed
but when we are silent
we are still afraid

So it is better to speak

– Audre Lorde

Prologue

T his book is a manifesto. I want to apply my suffering as a cancer patient and my life as a mother of a child with a disability as a springboard for social action. I am sharing myself with the distinct purpose of motivating positive change in the health care world. I hope the sparks of my story can ignite the revolution that begins with compassion both for those who are cared for and for those who are doing the caring. This is a book of a patient's wisdom about health care.

My intention is to not speak for other people who have had cancer, mothers who have children with disabilities or all those who work in health care. I especially do not represent people who have disabilities, for it is my son who is disabled, not I.

I am a woman of privilege. I have had many advantages in my life, being a white, university-educated, middle-class woman born in Canada, land of somewhat-socialized medicine. Despite all this, I still struggled to be heard as a patient and a caregiver. Imagine the other patients and caregivers. People themselves are not marginalized. People are people. It is society and systems that have been purposely built to include the gap of marginalization, to force space between those who have power and those who do not.

My combination of experiences as a patient, family member and

1

hospital employee are mine alone and I would not be so arrogant to believe that I could speak on behalf of others. There is no such thing as the voiceless. Other people do have a voice if we only take the time to listen.

I hope I can make a difference simply by telling my own story. I wrote this book to share how it feels to be a patient and a caregiver in the health system. I assert that compassion will blossom if people pause to try to understand another person's perspective. And the way that patients communicate about themselves is not through data or research. It is through stories.

Let this book be a crack for others to share their own stories to motivate, educate and inspire those who hold the power over us in the health system. As I continue to heal from cancer, may the telling of our stories help us all to heal – patients, families, staff and physicians alike.

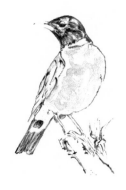

Hello
Health
Care

SUE ROBINS

My Rear View Mirror

∽ the beginning of my passion for health care ∾

The Good Girl

I was once in a workshop about broken people like me.
The grief counsellor said:
My story is my story.
And your story is your story.
And it is okay for them to be different.

People clutch their stories tightly, with white-knuckled hands.
Like purses stuffed with money in a late alley.

For instance, I have been told I should stay in my lane at all times.
Behave and be good. Do not be angry. Stay the rigid course.
And most of all be small in all ways.
If I step out of line, this rattles those who think they
own the story of me.

After I veer into my own way
The horns honk loudly before they slowly fade away.

– Sue Robins

I n my rear view mirror is a lifetime lived in health care. My
mother was a nurse. Her sister was a nurse. I was supposed to be
a nurse. My first job was at age 14, when I was paid to wash the toys

in the waiting room of a doctor's office. The next year, I graduated to candy striper, working Sundays as a volunteer on the extended care unit of a long-term care hospital. I brought patients down to a room at the end of the hall for church. The pastor arrived and the two of us sang together, off-key, "Jesus loves me, this I know, for the Bible tells me so." I helped feed lunch to old ladies who were cruelly tied into wheelchairs. Sometimes I just sat in the lounge, not knowing what to do, in a room full of patients, who were really just people. I held hands with paper-thin skin. Somehow just sitting by their sides in silence seemed enough.

When I was in Grade 12, I dutifully applied for a nursing degree program. I had good grades, even scooping up English and social studies awards in my quest to be perfect. I was a good girl, always seeking my parents' attention and approval. I applied to a university Bachelor of Nursing program and I was the first person in my family ever to go to university.

I was the epitome of the good girl. Nobody explicitly told me I should be a nurse, but I knew it pleased my family when I announced my intention to apply to nursing. I was carrying on a fine family tradition while ignoring what I truly loved, which were books and writing. For a solid 49 years of my life, many of the decisions that I made were an attempt to gain my family's approval. I finally gave up on all that when I got cancer.

I lost sight of myself in my quest to be perfect. I wonder how many young people choose certain paths in university so they do not disappoint their family. If they did have a burning passion, it eventually was extinguished in their attempt to be good girls and boys to make their family proud.

My parenting philosophy ended up being this: encourage your children to try all sorts of different activities when they are young, including sports, arts and academics. When they find the thing that makes them feel alive, support that thing unconditionally. While I do not regret my pit stop in nursing school, I do wish I had the confidence to unapologetically be myself. I'm half a century old and I'm still working on not making myself small.

A Lot of Heart

<curl> my struggle between compassion and professionalism <curl>

I'm not a mess. I'm a deeply feeling person in a messy world.
— *Glennon Doyle Melton*

Nursing education is a whole heck of a lot more about hard sciences than it is about the humanities. I encountered no art of nursing. In high school, I had been a stellar student in the arts. The heavy realities of statistics, anatomy and pharmacology nearly suffocated me in university. Nursing is tough in all ways and I am not.

I had hopeless technical skills, wincing before administering an injection, being ordered out of the Operating Room by a surgeon before I passed out on the sterile field. I had to take a walk around the hospital for fresh air after seeing a tracheotomy being changed on an elderly gentleman. Bodily fluids made me queasy and there were a lot of bodily fluids. A lot. I didn't have the stomach for nursing.

But it was more than even that. My heart bled all over my sleeve. I could feel the pain that others could feel. I was squeamish to inflict pain or watch pain being administered to others, even for good reasons. I irrationally thought, "That must hurt so much" as the surgeon cut into anesthetized patients. I was unable to turn that part of myself off. Nobody talked about this in nursing school, so I thought I was weak, fragile and the only one.

The truth is that good clinicians don't turn themselves off. They have compassion for themselves at the same time they have compassion for others. They allow themselves to feel the feelings instead of shoving their emotions into dark compartments. When feelings are shoved away, the pain always resurfaces, often in most unhealthy ways.

*I've come to believe that it's psychologically and spiritually damaging for a person **not** to be forcibly reminded of all the suffering in the world. – Chris Adrian* [1]

Health environments are filled with patients who are suffering. Health care professionals are not taught how to turn towards this suffering, so they often turn away instead. More suffering occurs when patient suffering is dismissed and minimized. This is how a vicious cycle is formed. Health care experiences can end up causing more trauma than the actual condition itself.

I still have no idea how my nursing classmates figured out how to grow a "thick skin" when witnessing or administrating painful procedures to patients. How I dearly wish my nursing instructors had spoken to us about how to help patients while taking care of ourselves. All the way through my hospital rotations, I always felt like my skin was peeled off. Nobody showed me how to feel compassion but not feel pain for patients.

I might have stayed in nursing if I'd had a mentor explain this to me. I needed to be taught how to process my own emotions around bearing witness to suffering. I wonder how many sensitive beings drop out of health care because of this lack of realization that it is okay to feel feelings at work. I thought I had to distance myself from patients so I could be protected from them. I was a fragile flower and I felt too much at every turn. At the age of 19, after having frequently been told I was overly sensitive, I thought I was deeply flawed. Today I know my sensitivity is a gift.

In my dreams, hospitals are healing environments for both patients and the people who work there. The concept of 'This is hard but important work' is discussed openly at reflective practice sessions together with patients, families and staff members. Debriefs, check-ins and space for listening are built into the workday.

This means that the notion of "what counts is counted" would need to be adjusted. Listening would count. Holding someone's hand would count. Offering a hug would count. Care would be administered human being to human being, not professional to patient. For once we break down the walls between roles and acknowledge that we are all human, well, that's the place where compassion is born.

Notes

1. Adrian, Chris. The Question, December 20, 2012, New England Journal of Medicine. https://www.nejm.org/doi/full/10.1056/NEJMp1212347

I'm Not Your Handmaiden

∽ experiencing moral distress in health care ∾

**Were there none who were discontented with what they have,
the world would never reach anything better.**

– Florence Nightingale

In my second year of nursing, I experienced a traumatic clinical rotation on labour and delivery. In the late 1980s, nurses were still shaving women's pubic areas and giving them enemas before carting them away to stark, brightly-lit operating rooms to give birth. This was before the days of soft lighting and wallpaper in labour rooms.

This routine shaving and giving enemas were all obstetric practice knew to do at the time. Later, research showed that these types of procedures are unnecessary and even harmful, and the shaving and enemas stopped. At the same time, women were asking for a more humane environment to have their babies. When I had my first child, a mere five years later, labour and delivery had evolved into a gentler place.

It is tough to break out of the "This is the way we have always done

13

it" mindset. Listening to patient feedback is a wonderful way to guide quality improvement initiatives. Back in the 1980s, the idea of improving the experience of the patient was just a pipe dream.

As a young student nurse, I was distraught at witnessing how the beautiful act of having a baby was stolen and medicalized for the hospital system's convenience. My good girl façade began to crack.

At that time, too, it seemed to me that nurses were handmaidens to doctors in the hospital. Only 20 years had passed from the era when nurses stood up when a doctor entered the room, as it had been in the 1960s. I prickled at being bossed around and having little autonomy beyond executing a doctor's orders.

I had not progressed far enough in my education to see that nursing autonomy was indeed present. At that time, in the late 1980s, nursing education requirements in Canada were being transformed from a two-year diploma program to needing a four-year university degree to enter nursing practice.

I found the weight of the system stifling. It was not until many years later that I realized that it is in an individual's control to make a difference, one patient at a time. Nurses do have power over how they treat and care for patients, even within the strict constructs of the hospital pecking order.

My second year in nursing I spent time on a pediatrics ward, where children of all ages were kept in cribs. They cried for their absent mothers all night long. This was the time of strict visiting hours and mothers were not allowed to stay overnight with their children, as this was the way that it had always been done. The sound of their crying still haunts me today.

In Praise of Nurses

∽ my gratitude for the nursing profession ↶

**To do what nobody else will do, a way that nobody else can do,
in spite of all we go through; that is to be a nurse.**

– Rawsi Williams

By my second year of nursing, it was becoming painfully obvious that I was not cut out to be a nurse. What it did do, though, was transform me into a person who is in awe of nurses and all that they do.

I can pluck out shining examples of good nurses over the years. My own mother, who worked at a nursing home, made sure to go to patients' funerals on her days off.

A friend shared a tender tale of going back to the Pediatric Intensive Care in the middle of the night, only to find a nurse sitting by her sedated son's bedside, reading him a children's book.

I once took an impromptu photo for an article I was writing of a licensed practical nurse carefully brushing the long hair of a woman who had dementia.

These above and beyond the call of duty stories are examples of how nurses make a positive impact every single day on patients and families' lives.

Nurses are often under-recognized, but they are truly the back-bone of the entire health system. They are uniquely the one profession that is with patients 24 hours a day, seven days a week. Patient care – and not just treatment – rests heavy on their shoulders. My last rotation in nursing was in orthopedics. This was the kind of unit I liked: the pace was less intense, and I could sit by a patient's bedside and chat. There were many patients there recovering from hip replacements and they moved slowly, like I did. Chatting with people was one of my favourite things to do. I was especially close to my own grandma, and I was fond of older people.

I had inadvertently stumbled upon the heart of health care in this last stage of nursing. The heart is demonstrated by actions like the comforting, the listening and the sitting by the bedside. I had excellent bedside manner, but in the era of counting costs, one tissue at a time, what was treasured in health care was efficiency, not kindness. I was not a fast nurse.

At age 19, I had no idea how to take care of my own heart, for I only knew how to give myself away to care for others. The realization that self-care has less to do with bubble baths and more to do with self-love has only appeared to me recently in the past few years. Nursing required a quiet kind of confidence that I did not possess.

Reflective practice was not a tool that was discussed in my two years of nursing school back in the 1980s. I know times have changed and there is more adoption of reflective practice activities in health care settings. Having the opportunity to debrief in a safe environment after something difficult happened would have helped me tremendously as a student nurse. Taking care of the caregiver – whether they are paid or unpaid – is absolutely necessary so they can go forth and take care of the patients.

In the end, I realize that I would have made an excellent church lady who visited members of the congregation who were hospitalized. If I had been luckier, I could have been guided into a profession like spiritual care or counselling that might have better suited my talents.

Because of my failures in nursing, I admire nurses very much. The best nurses possess a unique combination of the head and heart, the art and science, the left brain and right brain. I bow and tip my hat to all nurses.

Half a Nurse

∼ my final failure as a nursing student ∽

Staff culture eats patient centred care for breakfast.

– Me

Before I finally gave up, I soldiered on in nursing, loathe to be
a quitter. I even started to master more technical tasks. One
day a young man who had a terrible work-related accident praised
me for my gentleness while I changed his complex dressing. I was
gentle because I was careful and did not want to inflict more pain
on someone who had already experienced so much pain. I was
slow and methodical and I made sure to offer him pain medication
before I started. I had a sense that I would be a good nurse if I wasn't
rushed. Rushing caused me to focus solely on the task, not the patient. Thankfully, student nurses are given a lighter patient load and
usually I was gifted with time.

One particular day on orthopedics, I was assigned an older lady
who had an amputation from a complication due to diabetes. She
was a seasoned patient and she helped me through my assignment:
to wrap her stump, the remaining part of her amputated leg. This
required careful application of the bandage, a complicated figure
eight of a dressing that I applied and then reapplied until the ban-

dage was snug and sat flat.

"How does it feel?" I kept inquiring. "Fine, dear," she answered.

Later, I was in the staff room when the nurse I was partnered with came in the room to seek me out. I could see from the look on her face that I was in big trouble.

"WHO DRESSED MRS. S'S STUMP?" she yelled, looking at me, knowing full well the answer to her own question. I was meant to confess.

"Me," I squeaked out, standing up. "IT WAS TOO TIGHT! DON'T YOU DEGREE NURSES KNOW HOW TO DO ANYTHING?" she responded.

I scurried out of the room, red-faced with shame to right my wrong. Sure enough, Mrs. S's stump was indented with the marks of my too-tight bandage. I had screwed up. I carefully re-wrapped it, this time loosely just to be sure.

I could accept my rookie error. I apologized to Mrs. S, who was untroubled and forgiving. What I could not swallow was being yelled at. The only person who had ever yelled at me before was my own mother. Was I about to enter a profession where I was to be regularly yelled at?

At that moment, I had an odd combination of conviction about how I should be treated (as in: Nurses eat their young? They aren't eating me), along with my soft, sensitive heart. Being yelled at was not in alignment with my view of what I wanted for my life.

I marched over to the Student Centre to fill out the requisite forms to transfer far away from nursing to the other side of campus. Soon I was safely sitting in a classroom happily absorbing lyrical sonnets.

My parents, a nurse and plumber, were not thrilled about my decision to leave nursing. I had my university tuition cut off and in retaliation, I furiously moved out of their house one hot July afternoon. I had a boyfriend (and future husband) who was a musician in the arts program. Transferring out of nursing and hooking up with an "artsy-fartsy" were the greatest acts of rebellion a good girl could do to her parents.

I still got that damn university degree, but just a different one. Nobody yelled at me in English class, not even once, and that's the way I liked it. I emerged a few months later with a degree in Shakespeare and art history – the furthest thing from a health faculty degree that I could imagine.

I lasted exactly two years in that four-year nursing program. This later led to a running joke that I was half a nurse. I sort of know what to do in first aid situations and to this day can make a bed with sheets tucked in tight hospital corners.

Eat Your Young

~ how poor hospital culture can harm ~

**Failure is an imperfect word because the second you
learn from it, it ceases to be a failure.**

– Brené Brown

U npacking my half-nursing experience, I find a number of
important points. I do not believe that our nursing faculty
prepared us young pups for the reality of the hospital environment.
We were just thrown in and expected to swim.

I didn't expect to be sheltered, as this is patronizing, but I would
have appreciated some warning as to the political atmosphere in
the hospital. This was a harsh environment to be thrown into at a
tender age. It was a particularly hostile time in the staff room when
diploma-educated two-year Registered Nurses (RNs) were pitted
against nurses with four-year university degrees. They thought we
thought we were better than them and they did not hesitate to put
us in our place.

This was the beginning of my realization that health care is rife
with power struggles at all different levels: the classic doctor to
nurse, and then a complicated foray into the pecking order of nursing. Today most RNs with diplomas have retired and the majority of

nurses have their Bachelor of Science in Nursing degrees, but there are still many layers of conflict between nurses. The fighting to define who is a nurse and who is not continues to this day.

The hierarchies in hospitals are rampant and continue way beyond nursing: general practitioner v. specialist, union v. non-union, intern v. resident. I once sat on a panel with a selection of health professionals representing their regulatory bodies. Each of these professionals was squabbling about their own profession's scope of practice. When it was my turn to talk, I asked, exasperated, "Can't you all agree to get along in the sandbox, at least for the good of the patient?" I might be naïve, but I knew how this squabbling negatively affected patient care.

With all this fighting for power, not one drop of power drips down to the poor patient, who is left lying vulnerable and exposed on a hard hospital bed.

Thirty years later, with many unwanted glimpses into the health system, I can say that I wish there were 'softer' nurses out there. Nursing school either ate you up or spat you out. If you couldn't figure out your own boundaries, there was no middle ground. This inner work was beyond me in my early years.

Today, there is a lot of awareness about abusive behaviour in the workplace between colleagues, and many an anti-bullying campaign has been launched. Being yelled at in the staff room by another nurse was not okay in 1988 and it isn't okay now. But this type of insidious culture remains in health settings, fed by power structures and disdain of those considered weak, including young vulnerable students and patients too.

I've always believed that if morale is low among staff, then patient care will suffer. I do not think a nurse who just got yelled at in the staff room will walk into a patient's room and deliver safe and confident patient care as her morale slowly erodes away. I don't imagine those doing the yelling are particularly kind or compassionate towards their patients, either. If health professionals have such disdain for the weak, how does this translate into empathy for vulnerable patients?

Shakespeare in White Nylons

∽ my most important job: a nursing attendant ∾

You do not have to be good.
You do not have to walk on your knees
for a hundred miles through the desert, repenting.
You only have to let the soft animal of your
body love what it loves.
Tell me about despair, yours, and I will tell you mine.

– Mary Oliver

After transferring into the English program at the same university, my two years of nursing education helped me secure a part-time job as a nursing attendant in a veteran's home. I liked this job because I spent time with patients, helping them get up in the morning and assisting with breakfast. I liked to chat while I did my daily tasks, even if the patient wasn't able to respond. I would often show up at 7 a.m. for half an early morning shift and then run across campus in my white uniform and nylons to attend my Shakespeare classes.

Nursing attendants are true bedside workers. We were the ones who worked directly with the all-male patients on the nursing unit – many of whom required extensive care. We cleaned up things that the housekeeping staff wouldn't touch. We also had the luxury of time to spend with the veterans, as we helped them get dressed, or patiently helped feed them meals.

Nobody at the veterans' home talked about the war. At the time, there was even a World War I veteran living there – but most of the veterans were from World War II and Korea. While the war was in the distant past, it lived with these men every day. These were just ordinary men who had found themselves in terrible circumstances. The scars from those wartime experiences often were manifested in estranged families, whispers of abusive behaviour and alcoholism. I remember helping men to bed after their return from the pub, reeking of whisky and slurring their words.

But that wasn't the whole story. The wars had affected a cross-section of the population of men, and there were many dignified residents at the veteran's home. They enjoyed the company of the young nurses who were there to support them, and many of the patients reminded me of my own grandpa. It was important for the staff to remember that these 'patients' were also fathers, granddads, brothers and sons.

My clearest memory was one winter when I was working nights. On night shift, we sat at the nursing desk, waiting to respond to call bells. Every few hours, we would have rounds, where we would quietly walk through the unit, checking on the men, emptying urinals, and turning those who were immobile so they wouldn't get bedsores.

This particular night, my patient assignment included an elderly man named Harry. He was in the last stages of life, and his breathing was increasingly noisy and laboured. He had no family or friends to visit him in his final hours. After our first set of rounds, I excused myself from the desk to sit beside his bed. Harry had yelled and sworn at me in the past, but all that didn't matter now. His hand had paper-thin skin, and I held it softly through the wee hours of the night. It was a long shift. When I left at 7 a.m., I said a quiet good-bye and gave him a gentle kiss on his forehead. I did not look back when I left the room.

I was off for the rest of the week and read Harry's obituary in the paper a few days later.

I learned many things from working at that vet's home. One was to duck fast if something was being thrown at you. The other was that health care is really about acts of kindness. No person should ever die alone.

Cold Calling Nurses

∽ my start in health care administration ᔓ

There are years that ask questions and years that answer.
– Zora Neale Hurston

A fter I graduated with my English degree, I continued to work in health care. I may have failed to become a nurse, but I remained fascinated with health care. I was comfortable working in hospitals. I understood their general geography and mode of operation.

The elements of all hospitals are the same: admitting, gift shop, outpatient clinics, inpatient units, cafeteria. I soon discovered that there were other jobs in the hospital besides being a doctor or a nurse.

In 1989, there was no such thing as an automatic job for an English graduate. This is possibly true today too! But the joy of a liberal arts degree is that you can craft a career simply from being curious about new experiences and people.

At age 21, I got a job as a staffing clerk. This was a strange position that is mostly automated now. I had to get up at 5 a.m., drive to the hospital and call nurses to ask them if they could come into work to replace those who had called in sick. I had only a piece of paper and a telephone. I am an introvert and had always been terrified of talking on the phone. This job did not cure my phone phobia, but I had many amusing conversations waking up husbands at 6 a.m. and asking for their wives to see if they were able to work a day shift.

"My wife isn't here right now. I don't know when she's coming back," I was often told, overhearing the wife in question frantically whispering in the background.

I was the worst kind of cold caller. The group of nurses who worked casually was called the float pool and I quickly learned that people were generally unhappy being called at 6 a.m. They either wanted more work or less work – I could not seem to offer them the exact right amount of shifts.

This was the beginning of my recognition of how important relationships are in health care – all relationships – from clerk to nurse to patient. Relationships work all ways, starting from the lowest paid position on up.

If I did not have a good relationship with the nurses in the casual pool, they would not be motivated to come into work when I called them. If they did not feel valued, they would eventually become unhappy or simply leave. At my tender age, I was starting to understand how relationships were mutually beneficial. Plus, I was good at getting to know people. When nurses came to sign in for their shifts, we'd chat about our respective weekends. We started to get to know each other as people, not just as a clerk and a nurse.

I moved into a job at another hospital as a part-time unit clerk, secretary and staffing coordinator. It was a small hospital, one that housed tuberculosis, spinal cord injury and polio patient units. The basement had creepy tunnels that connected us to the acute care hospital across the street. The tunnels were lined up with dusty iron lungs, some of them child-sized, reminding me of the barbaric treatment of polio from the past. Today these patients would live in rehabilitation or long-term care facilities (or hopefully their own homes). This was the early 1990s when residential hospital living was still a thing.

This hospital was littered with security guards or police officers who often accompanied patients to the business office. They were assigned to patients who were incarcerated and had experienced a spinal cord injury. There were also patients with tuberculosis, many from Indigenous communities, who had guards to force them to stay in the hospital so they would take their medication. The security presence was heavy-handed and disconcerting. It was a stark reminder that some patients had no choice at all. Medicine knows best.

I learned a lot, including that the first order of business was always to make your boss look good. (This lesson stands true today, which is why I like to work for myself). My boss was the Director of Nursing, a terrifying old-school nurse who wore expensive shoes. I remember being hauled into her office and yelled at, though I can't recall what I exactly did. The sound of the click, click, clicking of her heels in the hallway instilled fright into the hearts of all the staff. We'd scurry off and hide in patient rooms if we heard her impending approach.

I soon discovered it was the unit clerks who actually run the nursing unit. Administrative support staff can hold a surprising amount of power, and set the tone for patients, staff and families. This was when I first realized how important first impressions are. If a unit clerk has his or her head down and looks up with a scowl at someone standing at the desk – well, the whole health care interaction is not off to a good start. The way in which staff welcomes patients affects their entire experience.

My meandering through junior roles in the hospital was useful. Nursing attendants are the lowest-paid positions of all the clinical roles. My perspective from the bottom showed me that hierarchies in hospitals run deep. Interestingly, the jobs with the least status, like receptionists and porters, often have the most patient contact.

If you are on the bottom of the pecking order and not treated well by those above you, you may end up taking out your frustrations on the people under you – who are patients.

These jobs proved to me this old adage: if you want an insight into someone's personality – to catch a glimpse into someone's character – watch how they treat a server in a restaurant. The same is true in the hospital. How the cashier in the cafeteria is treated by other staff is a litmus test that shows the culture in a hospital environment. I have never forgotten what it feels like to have started at the bottom.

My Black Business Suit

~ my transformation from health bureaucrat to mother ⌒

**Life is amazing. And then it's awful. And then it's amazing again.
And in between the amazing and the awful it's ordinary and
mundane and routine. Breathe in the amazing. Hold on through the
awful. And relax and exhale during the ordinary. That's just living
heartbreaking, soul-healing, amazing, awful, ordinary life.
And it's breathtakingly beautiful.**

– L.R. Knost

T hrough the rest of my 20s, I crawled up the health administration ladder. All of a sudden, it was the 1990s. I had traded in
my white nylons and starched nursing uniform for black pantyhose
and a black business suit with padded shoulders. I drove downtown,
feeling important in my now-corporate position with the Ministry
of Health. I flew around the province presenting with a co-worker
about funding formulas. This was a funny job for me, a person who
struggled both with math and public speaking. I stood in hospital
bathrooms with my co-presenter as we furiously rolled lint brushes
over our dark suits before we climbed up on the auditorium stage.

We often presented to crowds of hostile physicians, who did not appreciate us people from the health ministry. I was 22 years old and this was a hell of an introduction to public speaking.

This project work suited me. In between projects, I had gotten married to my first husband – the musician whom I had met in university – and I started having babies. I went off and on maternity leave, picking up projects along the way. After my first child was born, a beloved boy named Isaac, I left my maternity leave to return to a job in health care funding while my husband became a stay-at-home dad.

Health care funding is about as far away as you can get from patient care. Our project was about what I termed, counting Kleenexes – determining what resources were used in a hospital for patients with particular diagnoses. The more resource-intensive the patients, the more hospitals got paid. Previously, hospital budgets were assigned willy-nilly, for purely political reasons, depending on what constituency the hospitals were located in. The new funding formula guaranteed more equity for hospitals, but also favoured large urban hospitals with more complex patients and did nothing to provide incentives for keeping patients well. This bias towards funding Intensive Care Units instead of primary care is still alive in Canada today.

I became a patient only when I birthed my children. The first time, in 1993, I was a terrified first-time mom, pressured into an epidural and a subsequent forceps delivery of my 9-pound bundle of joy Isaac, who arrived with bruises on his face (sorry, Isaac, for that). I had three years of motherhood under my belt when Ella was born. I vowed to avoid the forceps disaster by being able to feel when I was pushing. In 1996, that meant declining the epidural, which completely numbed mothers from the waist down. (Today's epidurals do allow for some feeling).

Ella arrived two weeks early and so terribly fast that I didn't even have time to ask for pain control. She slid out of my body under the influence of no medication and with no forceps. Her unexpected natural birth fed directly into my anti-medical intervention philosophy that I had picked up when I was a student nurse in the labour and delivery ward a decade before. The experience was exhilarating.

In figuring out my own identity as a mother, I eschewed the traditional medical model to become a granola mom. I was a fan of the attachment parenting philosophy. I birthed my kids as naturally as I could, breastfed them a long time and carried them around in slings. They also did not watch television and to this day, my daughter points out that she knows none of the cultural references that come from watching Teletubbies or Barney.

I had no use for health care aside from dutifully vaccinating my children and taking them for basic check-ups. Without a crystal ball, I had no idea how fortunate I was to have so-called typically developing children during my first 10 years of motherhood.

A Rabid Breastfeeder

∽ sharing life lessons from motherhood ✐

The way we talk to our children becomes their inner voice.

– Peggy O'Mara

In the 1990s, attachment parenting was all the rage and breast-feeding went along with it. Dr. William Sears was the new Dr. Spock and I took the mantras from his Baby Book very seriously.

Dr. Sears has since fallen out of vogue for various reasons, but at the time, he was da bomb for me. Motherhood taught me that women's health and child health are intertwined. I gave my babies unconditional love because I did not grow up with unconditional love. I chose to mother in a different way than I was mothered. I rejected the spanking and the critical parenting that was a corner-stone of the 1970s.

Somehow, deep inside me, I knew that I wanted to attach strongly to my children when they were small so that they felt secure grow-ing up for the inevitable day that I would set them free. This meant that I carried my babies in slings, breastfed them when they were hungry, comforted them when they cried and held them until they fell asleep. There is not only one way to parent, but I was firm in my conviction to parent my way.

I also gravitated towards La Leche League, a non-profit organization that promotes breastfeeding. There are many things that mothers involved with La Leche League get out of their experience. For me, this was a women's group of like-minded moms. It was my version of a left-leaning mom's group for those who wanted to give breastfeeding a good go. It was at La Leche League that I first stumbled on the value of peer support – which to me simply means connecting moms together so they can support each other. It means belonging to a community in a world where community is rare. This is good for health too.

La Leche's outlook fit into my philosophy and I did the training to become a La Leche League leader. I mostly enjoyed connecting with new moms but I did not do well with the politics of the organization, and only lasted a couple of years. I made wonderful friends over that time and learned a lot about relationships and how to facilitate an inclusive, welcoming group. I had a glimpse into the resiliency of women, as it was slowly dawning on me how damn hard it is to be a good mother.

I do love babies, but I especially love supporting other mothers. Until I found this mom's group, I was terribly lonely being at home with a little baby for nine hours a day. Other moms were good for my mental and emotional health.

Little did I know that I'd take these lessons from being a rabid breastfeeder into my unexpected second life, one that was built after the sudden collapse of my first marriage. One morning, on July 7, 2000, I became the single mother of two small children, who were three and six years old. My perfect family disappeared into thin air. I was broke, unemployed and distraught. Naturally, I packed my kids up and moved to Norway.

The Norwegian Cure

∽ how hard life experiences build character (I hope) ∽

**Here is the world. Beautiful and terrible things
will happen. Do not be afraid.**
– *Frederick Buechner*

N orway is the best country in the world for a broken heart. Its
citizens are reserved and solemn; it is where people wear
black and smoke furiously on the streets. It is the perfect place to
experience sorrow.

In July 2001, it had been exactly a year since my husband left me.
I was living in a prairie city with my two children. I managed to eke
out twelve months hanging onto the family home by a mash-up
of babysitting, caring for a friend who had MS and writing over-
wrought book reviews for the newspaper.

Legal fees were mounting from my separation and I could no
longer stave off the credit-collecting wolves. After selling the house
– and my entire white-picket fence existence – I had nowhere to live
and no steady income. I did what any reasonable mother would do: I
packed up my son and daughter, ages seven and four, and moved to
Bergen, Norway.

My reasoning worked like this: I had to run away but I couldn't leave my kids. So I took them with me on My Great Nordic Breakdown.

They say the geographical cure doesn't work because you can't get away from yourself. But I was fleeing from ghosts other than myself: my self-inflicted poverty, my well-meaning, advice-dispensing friends and my questionable suitors, which mostly included out-of-work actors and needy musicians. My head was spinning from all this white noise.

I had an opportunity to live with a Norwegian family I had met when they were living in Canada. I was to tend to their three children, along with my own, for room and board and $700 a month. This seemed like a reasonable plan while I got my head screwed on straight.

Four thousand miles away in Bergen, our little family lived in the attic of a house that was embedded in the side of Mount Floyen. The rain fell relentlessly on the roof of the attic. It was a really good place to be sad. Even in public I felt terribly alone, surrounded by people speaking a language that I didn't understand. I often found myself sitting in a restaurant called the Zupperia, woefully slurping fish soup.

The kids and I walked up and down the mountain to get to town. We encountered rats squished by Norwegian bicycles and I once acquired a slug on the inside of my hat, its slime streaked across my forehead. (My now-adult children still giggle at this memory). The kids played Lego and set fire to homemade paper boats in the backyard creek. The family owned a giant Schnauzer dog. That's where I learned my only Norwegian words – gå og legg deg (go lie down). Each Saturday, the kids would head into Bergen to spend their allowance on exotic-sounding candy. We adopted the civilized Norwegian habit of the Sunday family walk. I gave up on home schooling my willful kids, and one week we hopped a flight to London, where we browsed the Tate Modern and Shakespeare's Globe Theatre. What my children lacked in academics, they made up with a strange combination of walking, boredom, arts and culture.

In Norway, I learned to be alone without the easy distraction of difficult men or the drama of divorce. I also learned to eat again, having arrived as a shrunken version of my former self. I was introduced to the great pleasure of breaking bread over family meals of reindeer meatballs and pickled herring.

At night, I'd walk on the mountain paths in the dark. I listened to the only song I had with me – U2's *Beautiful Day*, on my Discman (it was 2001, remember). I listened to the lyrics, "What you don't have you don't need now" over and over again as gospel. Although I felt sick with anxiety for my unknown future, it was during these hikes that I slowly became stronger. The secret to get up any damned mountain in the pitch dark is to simply keep putting one foot in front of the other.

Five months later, my tourist visa long expired, I was ready to go back to real life. I had witnessed how much my kids had missed their dad and made the decision to follow him to another city where he had relocated for work. The job gods shone down on me a week after my return. In fact, more than just the job gods were looking after me, as three days after starting my new position, I met a guy who ended up being my dear second husband.

I was wary of dating again, but this man – named Mike – slowly won me over. He was funny, curious, and oddly for me, a computer guy. He was totally not my usual type. My usual type was the tortured artistic man. My new type ended up being a kind of nerdy, kind of cool guy who loved me and my children unconditionally.

Mike and I had four kids all together – my two plus his two children, all under the age of 10. We started living together in a noisy blended house and I became unexpectedly pregnant. Nine months later, I gave birth to a wee baby boy.

A few weeks later, I was standing in a doctor's office, no longer as a staff member or a person in a business suit, but as a tired mother with leaking breasts and a soft floppy baby. I was about to be immersed in health care once again, after a long 10 year break, but this time as a caregiver.

In that doctor's office, the trajectory of my already-messy life was about to change once again. I was looking down at the squiggly results of my baby's genetic test. Every cell in my newborn son's body had an extra copy of the 21st chromosome. Just like that, I became the mother of a child with Down syndrome.

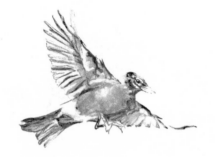

Welcome to Down Syndrome

The Baby You Expected is Not the Baby You Got

∽ in which we meet Aaron, the ⌣
baby who really wanted to be born

**I do not understand the mystery of grace – only that it meets us
where we are and does not leave us where it found us.**

– Anne Lamott

My baby boy was beautiful. He was the product of a second
marriage for both of us, evidence that broken people can
heal. He symbolized hope and joy. He was our love child.

Mike and I had been together just four months into our courtship
before I became pregnant. Aaron had unwittingly been conceived
two weeks before my husband had his scheduled vasectomy. We
already had two children each from previous marriages – this new
conception made us a family of seven. In retrospect and with a smile
on my face, I like to say that Aaron really wanted to be born.

His birth was everything I wanted. No interventions, no medications, a baby who slipped out naturally after a few pushes to meet

his parents. Even in the late stages of labour, Mike and I were giddy with excitement in between each contraction. "The baby is coming," Mike kept saying, and I would grin and nod and kiss my love before another wave of contractions pulled me back under.

We took him home after 10 hours, and he was all wee and jaundice-yellow. He was a quiet, soft, sleepy baby with a sweet mop of hair on top of his head. His round face was mine, and his eyebrows were blond. He was our little peanut, our button. His dad and I fell deeply in love with him.

Then the dark clouds started to settle in. At the end of his two-week checkup at the clinic, the doctor hesitated. I could tell he wanted to say something.

"Do you remember we talked about prenatal testing?"

Yes, I had. I had declined the testing. I knew I'd carry my baby to term no matter what.

I looked him straight in the eye, and took a deep breath. "Are you trying to tell me that our baby has Down syndrome?"

Retrospect is such an easy thing. I had not forgotten the day after Aaron's birth, when I had gotten up after a long night of scrutinizing my boy and typed "Down syndrome" in the Google search engine. I had broached the subject with Mike, and he had scoffed at me for being paranoid. Then I had asked the public health nurse later that day if she thought Aaron had Down syndrome.

"Yes," she had said gently, but then she had inspected the palms of his hands and his toes and concluded that he had a heart-shaped face like his mom, and eyes like his dad — that's all. No other signs. So we filed away this scare in the back room of our heads and carried on. Whew. That was a relief.

But when the doctor mentioned the prenatal testing, I knew. I could hear my heart beating in my ears. I was holding onto my baby for dear life. "Oh," I said. "Can I use my cell phone here?" I had to phone Mike, immediately.

I don't recall our conversation. I am sure I sounded as if I was being strangled — and, in a way, I was. I do know that I sat in that examining room, nursing Aaron until Mike arrived. I don't cry easily and there was a choked bundled of tears sitting just beyond my throat. I remembered to breathe.

Mike wanted to carry Aaron over to the lab in the hospital. He wouldn't put him in his stroller, and he marched proudly through the hospital corridors cradling his son. It was as if he was saying, "I'm looking after my boy, no matter what!" They drew blood from Aaron's little arm. Mike and I didn't talk much — I felt sick as the needle went in and Aaron gave a cry of protest. We had to wait two long weeks for the result.

We were back at home. Aaron was napping in his car seat. The day was beautiful...mid-April, sun streaming out of the prairie sky. We sat on the balcony of our house, watching Aaron sleep, discussed how our doctor was wrong, how he was too inexperienced, how he had surely misdiagnosed.

There was a waft of music coming from the house across the alley. I strained to make out what song it was — it was coming from an open bedroom window. A young man lived there with his parents. He had a rare chromosome deficiency and is one of the few people with such a condition to be alive. He wasn't expected to live beyond a year old, but there he was, 20 years old, blasting music out of his window.

The song finally became clear. It was a song from my memory of junior high school dances. Our neighbour was playing ABBA's *Take a Chance on Me*.

The results came back after the two weeks. And yes, our baby had Down syndrome. My deep chasm of grief seemed endless when we found out that the baby we expected was not the baby we received.

But slowly the sun peeked out from behind those clouds, and I was able to get out of bed and go about my business. My baby did not allow me to stay stuck in the grief, and neither did my husband. Mike and I had been through so much by this point, when we were told our baby had Down syndrome, my husband shyly smiled, shrugged and said, "Well of course he does."

At age two, Aaron held out his chubby little hand as we trundled down the sidewalk, both delighting in a warm fall day. My AB-BA-playing neighbour was outside as we passed his house, and his face lit up as I greeted him by name. Take a chance on us, indeed.

Sixteen years later, Mike and I steadfastly remain together, the love of each other's lives. Aaron was the early glue that sealed our deal.

A version this essay was originally published in the Globe and Mail, October 6, 2005.

Happy and Healthy Baby

~ explaining how it feels to have a baby born with a disability ~

Welcome to Holland.

– *Emily Perl Kingsley*

Aaron's Down syndrome diagnosis immersed me back into the world of health care in an entirely different way. I was no longer a candy striper, a student nurse, a nursing attendant, a unit clerk or a staffing coordinator, or a Ministry of Health bureaucrat.

I was brand new mom in the deep recesses of grief, holding a baby who I loved but who I did not understand. Everything I thought I knew about motherhood was gone too. My identity as a mom of two typically-developing children had been taken from me. I was instantly and involuntarily a special needs mom.

Every mother on earth wishes for a happy and healthy baby. But what happens if the baby you birth isn't healthy? Does that mean you've failed as a mother in your very first task of motherhood: giving birth?

Emily Perl Kingsley's *Welcome to Holland* essay is often shared with new families. It is a story of expecting to go to Italy – when you have

47

a typical baby – but ending up in Holland when you have a baby with Down syndrome instead. Kingsley has a son with Down syndrome and knows well the adjustment of getting used to a different land when a baby with an unexpected diagnosis is born.[1]

Babies are born early. Babies are born with medical conditions. Babies are born needing surgery. Babies are born with disabilities. These outcomes are rarely discussed in the world of expectant mothers. These are the secrets of motherhood, along with the pain of labour, postpartum depression and hemorrhoids. Nice people don't talk about such things.

In my sheltered world, I had never given one moment of thought to this, except briefly four years earlier when a dear friend gave birth to a son who was stillborn. It was a shock to privileged me that the natural order of life had been so disrupted by a little baby dying before he had lived. Even though I had spent my early career in health care, I still thought that these disruptions happened to other people, not to those I loved.

Other people had disabled children. With the addition of my son's extra 21st chromosome, I became the other. I was submerged into the mother of all identity crises.

For my third child, the concept that there's no such thing as a perfect child was taught very early, way before adolescence. For some families, it is as we blink back tears in the delivery room. This is difficult to process so early on in our stories, as we grapple with raging hormones, sleep deprivation and shock. But process it we must. We have not failed and our child has not failed. We've been turbo-boosted into the imperfect world of motherhood and we must now get to the work of loving our child.

We have no choice but to begin serious mothering when we have just freshly given birth to any child, whether they have a disability or not. Here's one thing that I don't think people understand about having a kid with a disability: we love all our children, no matter what. Your three-month-old won't sleep? Your toddler is screaming in the grocery store? Your 11-year-old is failing math? You do not stop loving your child. Your nine-year-old acquires a brain injury in a car accident? Your teenage daughter has an eating disorder? Your 20-year-old struggles with addiction problems? You do not stop loving these children either.

As children grow up, they surprise us, they shock us, they sadden us and they leave us. This is natural and normal. Everybody learns that there's no such thing as a perfect child when our children are teenagers. One day your child says he hates you, another day the principal calls.

Parenting is hard work, and that's how it should be. We have not failed in birthing our sweet, soft babies. We are thrust onto the bumpy road of mothering when we are least ready for it. We are inexperienced and fragile. We find out early that there's no such thing as perfect or normal. While most mothers bask in the innocence of their healthy children, we know different.

Aaron is different from us at the chromosomal level in his body. It took us some time to learn that he was like us too. As he grew up, we have seen the love of sports from his dad and his sensitive heart that was inherited from me, his mom. But I did not know all this when he was born. All I knew was fear. I was fearful of the other.

The skills we acquire in those dark early days serve us well as mothers. We understand that stuff happens, and that things do not always go according to plan. We carry that resiliency and flexibility forward into motherhood. We are but ordinary people doing extraordinary parenting. That doesn't seem like a failure to me.

Notes
1. Kingsley, Emily Perl, Welcome to Holland, 1987, http://www.our-kids.org/Archives/Holland.html

Sharing the News

~ stressing the importance of disclosing diagnosis well ~

**The trajectory of a whole family's life changes in the
moment a diagnosis is shared. So don't screw it up.**
— My advice to pediatric residents

W hen I was 12 weeks pregnant, my physician offered me
blood work for prenatal screening. He didn't describe what
the screening was actually for, but even as a naïve layperson, I knew
well enough that it was to test if the baby had Down syndrome. I
turned down the testing. To have or not have screening and subsequent testing is an intensely personal decision in any pregnant
woman's life.

At the end of Aaron's two-week appointment, I sensed that my
doctor was exceedingly uncomfortable. He was shifting his weight
back and forth and I remembered looking down at his shoes. He
wore brown suede ankle boots that were in style at the time, called
desert boots. I won't ever forget them.

It has been 16 years yet I can still recall where I was standing in
the room. In fact, I could see the whole clinic room, as if I was taking
an aerial picture from above. I know now that the sense of floating
above my body is a traumatic response. In this moment, my whole

life, my whole family's life, was about to change with the utterance of this young doctor's poorly-chosen words. I still feel the sharp sting of his question:

"Do you remember when we talked about prenatal diagnosis?"

What I heard when he asked that was, "Do you remember that we talked about aborting this baby?" Clearly, I had not aborted my baby. I was holding him in my arms. He was tiny, but very much loved, wanted and alive. It was the exact wrong way to introduce the notion of Down syndrome.

After dumping the diagnosis on me, my doctor then turned on his heel and abruptly left the room. I was alone there with my baby for the longest 20 minutes of my life. I remember sitting there, nursing my beloved boy, trying not to cry. I couldn't cry in front of my baby. What would it say to him that I was sad about him?

Travels in the world of health care often begin with the disclosure of a diagnosis. It has taken me years to forgive this family doctor who introduced the concept of my baby having Down syndrome through his prenatal testing comment. This is neither sensitive nor wise. Asking about prenatal screening and testing is a moot point once the baby is born. Many physicians and physicians-in-training have asked me about it throughout the years – including when Aaron is right there in the room. I now decline to answer. "What relevance does that have now?" I ask.

I knew my doctor was young. In fact, I had chosen him for that reason – a family physician to provide prenatal care so I wouldn't be bothered with unnecessary interventions during my labour. That part was effective – he had allowed me to labour unencumbered by IVs, catheters or Pitocin to speed up my contractions once my water had broken.

I know my doctor left me in the clinic room that day because he was uncomfortable and had other patients to attend to. I wish he hadn't left me all alone. Perhaps if he was in a hurry, he could have asked one of his team members – a nurse – to offer to sit with me in the room? This seems like a simple solution. Surely clinics can accommodate some extra time for patients and families who are there reeling from unexpected news? This is a pretty basic thing to do on the spectrum of kindness in health care. Could more than 10 minutes be allotted of a physician's time? It is important.

Two weeks later, the definitive results from Aaron's testing came in. The doctor called my husband on the phone to tell him the news that our baby did indeed have Down syndrome. My husband was driving at the time and had to carry that news with him throughout his work day, until later that evening when the kids were settled in bed. Then he had to tell me himself that our baby had Down syndrome.

Now, I wish there were things different about this diagnosis story. For about ten years, I was in a rage towards my doctor. You might call this shooting the messenger. It is true that I would have been unhappy with anybody sharing this unexpected news with me, but had it been shared in a less harmful way, we might have maintained a good relationship.

Having diagnosis disclosed in a positive way puts families in a place of strength, not devastation. In amongst my inevitable grief over the loss of a "healthy" baby, I could have drawn upon hopeful and positive words from our physician to help our family on our path of acceptance (and eventual celebration) of Aaron's Down syndrome.

The rest of my family saw the same family doctor for many years. My husband went to him and my older kids, too, for this doctor ended up specializing in adolescent medicine. We know he was well meaning, but inexperienced. I've come to understand that he just did not know how to handle disclosing our son's diagnosis to us.

I wish that the whole thing went down differently.

I wish when our doctor had first brought up Down syndrome, he had asked for both my husband and me to be at the appointment.

I also wish he hadn't mentioned prenatal testing when he talked about Aaron. Prenatal testing is an exceedingly sensitive issue to the Down syndrome, spina bifida and neural tube defect communities. It is crucial for health professionals to be aware of that.

It was unfair to pass the burden of telling me that our son had Down syndrome to my husband. Telling him on the phone, while he was driving, wasn't the right thing to do, either. Instead, I wish our doctor had booked a follow-up appointment two weeks after the blood test was taken to share the genetic results with both my husband and me in person.

Physicians often learn about how to disclose diagnosis from their mentors – the doctors they are training under when they are medical students, interns, residents and fellows. If their mentors are uncomfortable with this task, if they are rushed or use biased language, then the young doctors might be that way too.

A few years later, I presented about sharing the news to a group of pediatric residents. There were about 15 residents in the room and all of them happened to be female. I co-presented with a geneticist and she talked to them about how it feels for her to disclose diagnoses to families. It was so important to talk honestly about how difficult this task is for physicians, to open the door for the residents to share their own stories. By the end of our talk, we were all in tears, speakers and audience members alike.

The geneticist said some important things: she said even though she'd been in practice for 25 years, telling families unexpected news about their child is still the hardest thing she had to do. She said she honoured the gravity of what she was about to do by preparing beforehand: thoroughly reading the chart, sometimes bringing another colleague with her so she wouldn't be alone and by pausing and taking a deep breath before she knocked on the door of the hospital or clinic room. She also talked about debriefing with her team afterwards in order to take care of herself.

I watched in awe as this senior physician was vulnerable enough to be open about her feelings on stage in front of these students. We did a round-table exercise when we asked each of the pediatric residents about their experiences sharing news with families. Some had to tell families that their child had died in a car accident. Others gave cancer diagnoses. Others shared the results of genetic tests, as had happened with our family. It was then I realized how difficult sharing the news was on physicians too. It is a task that nobody wants to do and that is why it is often done poorly. I wonder if caring for the physicians before, during and after this challenging duty would help it go better for all those involved, including the patient and their family.

I can speak with mothers whose children with Down syndrome are grown up – now 30 years old – and they remember the day the news is shared with them like it was yesterday. We never forget.

There's No Such Thing as the Perfect Child

~ my commentary on the ethics of the prenatal testing question ~

...by gripping tightly to the story of good or bad, I close down my ability to truly see a situation.

– Heather Lanier

Over the years, I have been asked by medical students, other moms and even strangers if I had prenatal testing when I was pregnant with Aaron. I find it odd because what difference does the answer make now? Obviously, I carried my pregnancy to term, because there is my son, alive and well, standing right there beside me. The prenatal testing question is not only odd because it is irrelevant; it is offensive too.

A word to the wise for those wanting to ask a parent if they had prenatal testing: don't do it. What you are really asking us is, "Why didn't you abort your child?" And, similarly, "Why is this child even alive right now?" Justifying the very existence of our beloved children hurts. There is no medical reason to ask it, except for an intrusive kind of curiosity.

One day over a dozen years ago, a mom from my son's preschool class stopped me in the playground on the way to my car. I had handed out a letter that explained about my son's Down syndrome to the parents in the class. Families who have kids who are different often do this, in hopes of educating the other families about acceptance.

This mom chitchatted with me a bit and then said she was surprised by the letter. I responded that I was hoping if I explained about Aaron, it would help foster understanding.

Then she got to her point. She really wanted to know why I didn't get prenatal testing. Not if I got prenatal testing, but why I didn't get prenatal testing. The question veered way beyond curiosity right into a highly offensive zone.

I looked at her, puzzled. It seemed like a funny question to ask, and staggeringly inappropriate to boot, but I had been asked a version of it before – by medical students taking Aaron's history in the hospital and at a mom-and-baby yoga class when Aaron was only four months old. I felt the sting of that question every single time it was asked.

I thought, rationally, "Here's your chance to educate – I am an ambassador against ignorance." I answered her cheerily, "Well, testing wouldn't have changed my pregnancy outcome, so I turned the testing down."

Out of the corner of my eye, I could see my car in sight. It was my escape hatch, but it was several metres away. I had to immediately extract myself from this conversation because I felt as if I was floating above my own body.

I said my (pleasant) goodbyes and scrambled to my vehicle as fast as I could in the winter snow.

I slid into the driver's seat, slumped over the steering wheel and burst into tears. I'm not much of a crier. But it was as if I had been slapped.

I continued crying all morning in parking lots in between running errands. I cried in the coffee shop drive-through and in the grocery store lineup. I had to bite my lip to prevent the tears from falling down my face in public.

Why do I have to justify my son's very existence? Why isn't it okay that he's alive? What are you afraid of?

For those of us who have children whose extra chromosomes could have been detected prenatally, this questioning puts us on a long and lonely road. We get frantic calls from friends who are considering amniocentesis because their prenatal screening came back elevated. Then we are expected to celebrate with them when the results come back saying their baby doesn't have Down syndrome. "Hurrah, you aren't having a child like mine?"

The whole genetic testing thing is fraught for parents who have kids with disabilities. One day it won't just be families of disabled children dealing with this. With the clever mapping of genes, there may be tests for all the lovely imperfections of life that make us human, all in the quest for the blue-ribbon baby.

This isn't a pro-choice or anti-abortion issue. It is about the value of a human being. If mothers must be asked if they had prenatal testing, perhaps a gentler "Was your baby's diagnosis a surprise?" would be a better question to begin a conversation.

Point of Conception

~ dreaming of changing the way people see Down syndrome ⌒

**All parenting turns on a crucial question: to what extent parents
should accept their children for who they are, and to what extent
they should help them become their best selves.**

– Andrew Solomon

Down syndrome occurs at the point of conception. For Aaron,
he always had it. For me as his mom, my initiation into the
world of having a child with a disability was my new reality.

It was unusual for his diagnosis to come so late. Most Down syndrome diagnoses come prenatally or right in the delivery room. A
nurse or the physician will recognize something different about the
baby – low-set ears, almond-shaped eyes, a gap between the toes.
Sometimes, but not always, the baby has urgent medical concerns
that alert them in the direction of Down syndrome, like difficulty
breathing or a heart condition.

I'm not sure why nobody at the hospital picked up on Aaron's
markers for Down syndrome. Maybe it was because he was born at
12:30 in the morning and we only stayed for 10 hours. It could have
been because a resident caught him – I hesitate to say a resident
delivered him, as I was the one who delivered him through my own

sheer will! It probably was because Aaron had no serious medical complications, so nobody looked at him that closely. For me, not knowing he had Down syndrome for the first two weeks of his life was a good thing. I fell in love with him deeply as a person, without all the shock and readjustment that comes along with suddenly finding out you have a disabled child.

Some call this readjustment grief. My mantra continues to be that the baby I expected was not the baby I got. I had to grieve for the baby I expected in order to accept the baby I now had. Some people don't agree with this grief model but this was my reality. Every family is different.

If I'm truly honest, this adjustment had more to do with me and my own ego, misconceptions and ableist ideas about people with Down syndrome. I know that some health professionals grapple with these things too, for it comes through in how they handle sharing a diagnosis of disability and the subsequent care they provide for their patients.

This circles back to the question: who gets to decide who is human? What assumptions do health professionals have about people with disabilities and how do those assumptions harm patients and families?

My dream is one day news about Down syndrome is presented in the media, in novels, and by health professionals in the way news about twins is shared. As with any unexpected diagnosis, there is time for adjustment to accept the baby I have, instead the baby I thought I had. But there's no need to engage in fear mongering about Down syndrome.

Down syndrome has been around for a very long time – perhaps from the beginning of human history. Images of people with this chromosomal difference have been identified from the 15th century. Since I've been Aaron's mom, I've thought a lot about the meaning of disability. I believe that people with disabilities are a part of the human fabric, just like all other people with differences. In fact, many of us will experience disability ourselves in our lifetime. The phrase, "We are all one car accident away from a disability," reminds us we are all vulnerable to unexpected news in our lives.

I had the experience of visiting a family who had just adopted a baby girl with Down syndrome. The baby's name was Emily. Emily's mom was beaming when she answered the door. She and her husband were thrilled to have their long-awaited daughter in their arms. We talked about resources and services, but mostly we just basked in the joy of that new little girl. Emily was very much wanted and loved.

Contrast that with the way most biological families receive a diagnosis of Down syndrome. If it is a prenatal diagnosis, clinicians can set up automatic appointments for termination, and use terminology like "burden" and "suffering." After birth, families are often shunted away to rooms at the end of maternity wards. Hospital photographers never show up to take baby photos. Nurses avoid the room and social workers peek in the window. Nobody brings flowers or balloons. Hardly a celebratory welcome to the world for that beautiful new baby. The birth of every single baby deserves to be celebrated, and what health professionals sometimes forget is that most of us parents love our children unconditionally.

Andrew Solomon has written a wonderful book called *Far From the Tree*. It is ground-breaking work about children who are different from their parents. He extensively interviews families with children who are deaf, or born with dwarfism or who have Down syndrome like Aaron. He draws parallels with his own experiences being a gay man and searching for approval from his own parents.[1]

> *Rumi said that light enters you at the bandaged place. This book's conundrum is that most of the families described here*

have ended up grateful for experiences they would have done anything to avoid. – Andrew Solomon

How I wish all authors, journalists, editors and health professionals would read Solomon's book to understand that different is not bad. It is just different. Even if you do see having a baby with a disability as a tragic event, don't transfer your subjective values onto your readers and families.

Saying "Congratulations" instead of "I'm sorry" would go a long way to contributing to progressive change in this world. I might have stars in my eyes, but I hope for a world where we all belong, disability or no disability. It is within our own individual power to make this happen.

Notes

1. Solomon, Andrew, Far From the Tree: Parents, Children and the Search for Identity, 2012, http://andrewsolomon.com/books/far-from-the-tree/

About Dr. Darwish

∽   meeting our beloved pediatrician,   ⌒
who shows us the true meaning of kindness

Health care is two separate words: health and care.

– The rules of grammar

D r. Azza Darwish had a very busy pediatric practice. I first called
her office when Aaron was three weeks old. The receptionist
immediately booked us into a spot at noon the next day. When my
husband and I arrived at the clinic, I realized that they were actually
closed for lunch. I was grateful to sit in the quiet waiting room, and
not be surrounded by seemingly typical babies. That would have
been difficult in the fragile early days of Aaron's diagnosis. I was living under a heavy black veil of grief, where everything was very dark.
I did not wish to have happy gurgling babies obstructing my view.

We were escorted back to Dr. Darwish's treatment room. Mike
carried Aaron, who was asleep in his car seat bucket. The clinic
room was full of photos of Dr. Darwish's patients – kids with facial
differences, kids in wheelchairs, typical looking kids, and yes, I
recognized the heart-shaped faces of children with Down syndrome.
The display was a beautiful celebration of all the diverse children in
her practice.

We perched anxiously in our chairs, not talking. I picked nervously at my fingers as Mike stared at the ceiling.

Soon after, Dr. Darwish knocked on the door, came in and introduced herself. The very first thing she did was scoop slumbering Aaron up out of his car seat and held him in her arms. Today, 10 years later, I still can close my eyes and recall this well-dressed physician cuddling my son. It was a powerful image.

"You have a beautiful baby boy," she said, and a lovely smile spread across her face.

In the weeks after Aaron's diagnosis, we visited many health professionals. Not one of them held Aaron. Not one of them commented on how beautiful he was. And he was indeed beautiful – wee, soft, a bit floppy, with a mess of dark, punk-rock hair. Dr. Darwish was the first clinician to see Aaron as a baby first. She didn't immediately zero in on what was wrong with him. She first saw, and expressed, what was right.

She continued chatting with us, "It must have been quite a shock for you to find out about the Down syndrome." This opened the door for us to talk about how we felt about Aaron's diagnosis. Again, not one other clinician had asked us how we were emotionally. They all talked about risks, statistics and data. Nobody focused on what was invisible to the eye.

Our appointment was close to an hour long. I knew that was almost unheard of in the world of specialists. Dr. Darwish asked us if we wanted to see some of Aaron's physical markers. We did. She gently pointed them out. She carefully opened Aaron's hands, as if to read his palm. She softly showed us his lower-set ears and the gap between his toes. She murmured to him as she completed her examination. He was not a lab specimen to her. She treated him with such dignity, as if he was her own child. Over a decade later, my eyes still well up recalling this kindness.

Dr. Darwish patiently explained all the services available to us, and suggested we get in touch with our local support group so we could meet other families. She said her office would look after all the medical referrals we needed – for an echocardiogram and ECG, for audiology and ophthalmology. She made an overwhelmingly difficult experience more manageable, and ultimately, more human.

When we left her clinic, the waiting room was starting to fill up with patients for their 1 p.m. appointments. When we passed by Dr. Darwish's office, I could see her sitting at her desk, unwrapping her bagged lunch. She had spent her entire lunch hour with us – and we were a family she didn't even know.

Azza Darwish passed away from cancer 14 years ago. She was 52 years old. She is sorely missed in our community because of her skill as a clinician, as she had many children with Down syndrome in her practice. But she is mostly missed because of her compassion as a human being. She was a beloved pediatrician.

I cannot overstate the importance for health professionals to give patients and families the gifts of compassion and hope. After that appointment with Dr. Darwish, my heavy black veil of grief began to lift, ever so slightly. From beneath that veil, I caught my first real glimpse of my little boy. He continues to shine his light brightly on us today. Thank you, Azza, for this gift.

A version of this essay was originally published in the Canadian Medical Association Journal, May 2014. This is shared with kind permission from Dr. Darwish's husband, Alaa Elwi.

My Ego in an Orange-Striped Turtleneck

~ on stereotypes and the value of hope ~

**If you are going to have a stereotype, at least make sure it
is an up-to-date stereotype. Don't tell me about the boy with
Down syndrome you saw in church thirty years ago.**

– Monica S.

When Aaron received his Down syndrome diagnosis at two
weeks old, I was covered in a blanket of fear. The thought of
my baby having Down syndrome chilled me to the bone. There was
my baby, who I loved, but more than anything, I did not want the
Down syndrome. I did not yet know that Down syndrome is a part of
Aaron like my green eyes and curly hair are a part of me. Genetics
run deep. But Down syndrome made me uncomfortable as hell.

I had an image of a person with Down syndrome embedded in
my head. It was someone with a bowl haircut, large glasses and an
orange and brown striped turtleneck. This stereotype came from a
memory of walking past a special education school when I was about

11. I could see kids playing in the fenced-off playground and must have caught a glimpse of a young boy with Down syndrome in the orange striped turtleneck. This stayed with me.

What is especially ridiculous about this image is that the year must have been 1979. Everybody had a bowl haircut, big glasses and an orange striped turtleneck back then. But my idea of what someone with Down syndrome looked like was frozen in a stereotype in time.

It is the responsibility of those disclosing diagnoses to have a sense of what life with that diagnosis is really like. This goes beyond text-books; this means talking to other patients and families and listening to their stories.

A few years ago, I was at a pre-admission clinic before minor surgery. I was asking the doctor a lot of questions, wanting definitive answers. He said something that stayed with me.

"There is no such thing as always or never in medicine."

While patients might demand that you have a crystal ball, and while it might be tempting to say you have an answer to everything, the real facts of life mean that nobody knows anything for sure. However, it is helpful to understand the wide range of variations in between always and never.

For instance, telling people they will never walk after they have a spinal cord injury is mostly harmful. So is telling me that my son will always live with me. Who knows if either of those things will be true? Knowing and communicating the range of possibilities is important.

Disability is where we veer off-course of our carefully planned life. There must be nothing more horrifying to a doctor than a patient who cannot be cured, especially a baby.

Here we wade into the territory of health professional values. Hope does not mean a cure; hope can simply mean hope for a better day. Just because you think having a child with a disability would be a terrible thing for you, is it fair to assume that all families feel that way? And how can you be 100% positive about how you would feel at the time?

True, if you asked me when Aaron was first born, I would have said that Down syndrome was bad news. But within a few months, I started to realize that his extra chromosome was integral to him being Aaron, just like my own genetic makeup makes me who I am. Assumptions are killers – it is best not to make them and deliver news in a value-neutral way. Allow families and patients to place their own values on the news, in their own time, instead.

Second Circle of Diagnostic Hell

∽ the importance of making time to do the good work ∾

**Any parent of a child with a syndrome remembers
the day he or she is told to see the genetics department.
It is the second circle of diagnostic hell.**

– Ian Brown

I think a lot about the time when our son was first diagnosed. Us families never forget. We had many referrals to clinics and appointments with health professionals. I recall nothing about those times, except the extreme examples of mistreatment, and on the other end, the rare occurrences of kindness. Words matter and how our children are treated matters too. We are watching closely.

I remember the geneticist who stood gathered with students around my little baby, and how she treated him like a scientific specimen. She blandly described all his physical markers for Down syndrome like Aaron was a dissected frog. I glared at this geneticist, unable to even speak. This was our second circle of diagnostic hell.

Once I co-presented with another mom at a medical genetics clinic about the value of connecting parents for peer support. We both had children with Down syndrome, then ages five and 8, and we included pictures of our children in our PowerPoint.

There was an older male geneticist at the back of the room. I could see that he was visibly agitated during our presentation. Oddly, audience members forget that speakers can see them as we are speaking. Finally, during the question and answer portion of the talk, he burst out:

"What happens when your children aren't cute anymore?"

My co-presenter and I stood there in stunned silence. He continued to rattle on about all the burdens carried by people with Down syndrome when they were adults. We let him speak. He was digging his own grave in a room full of his colleagues.

If I had been quicker on my feet when he said, "What happens when your children aren't cute anymore?", I should have retorted, "What happened when you weren't cute anymore?"

This was a man who disclosed, on a regular basis, a diagnosis of Down syndrome to families, both pre and postnatally. How value neutral could his disclosure be if he harboured such anger and disgust towards adult people who had Down syndrome? Later, a genetic counselor called me to apologize. It was too late. I'd already had a glimpse into his dark world.

I have since met other geneticists who were of a gentler heart. I do not wish to dismiss an entire specialty, but it is important to point out the profound effect one person can have on another person's life, particularly if they are interacting with patients and families when they are in terribly vulnerable situations. Genetic counsellors seem to understand the relational subtleties of their work. Life is not black and white; nor is genetics a pure science – as when dealing with human beings, there are many shades of grey.

The evolution of kindness is empathy, and the demonstration

of empathy is compassion. The number one thing that health care needs right now is more compassion. Compassion for themselves and each other as health care professionals is important. Equally important is compassion for the patients and their families that they have signed up to serve and care for. That would be a good start.

And yet, patients are not mind-readers. They will never know that you care about them unless you show them. There must be a demonstration of compassion, something that reaches from one person to another. The showing of compassion can look like this: a hand on a shoulder, a kind word, a gentle tone. Kindness does not take more time.

I attended a profound presentation from researcher and nurse Dr. Betty Davies about "Best Practice Health Providers" at an ethics lecture. She spoke about creating space to actively listen to patients to find out what really matters to them. Afterwards, an audience member stood up and announced:

"We don't have time to do all this. We are too busy."

He was too busy to listen to patients? This is a common response to pleas to be more kind, slow down, create space for patients. The lecturer paused and looked down. I knew she had encountered this question before.

I will never forget when Dr. Davies raised her head and slowly said, "It doesn't take longer to hang an IV with a smile than with a frown." Then she explained that best practice health providers don't take time to do this work; they make time to do this work.

The Wonder

∿ insight into the joy Aaron has brought to our family ∿

I believe, fate, fate smiled

Destiny laughed as she came to my cradle

Know this child will be able

Laughed as my body she lifted

Know this child with be gifted

With love, with patience, and with faith

She'll make her way.

– Natalie Merchant

My youngest son is now 16 years old. The trajectory of our entire family's lives changed when his doctor uttered the words Down syndrome.

Years have passed and the intense grief has faded. I've realized that there is loss associated with parenting all children. No child is perfect and all children are hard work. But with typically developing children, we learn this lesson gradually as they grow up. With our kids with Down syndrome, we are told this immediately upon diagnosis. For me, it felt as if I had been hit by a truck.

We must honour the healing that comes from the dark times. For many months, I was mourning the loss of the so-called perfect baby. Looking back, there were many factors that helped me move forward to see the light again.

My personality is good for people – for love – like my family.
– Aaron

Having Aaron in our lives has changed our entire family. He has infused all of us with wonder. His two older siblings were six and nine when he was first born. His sister Ella, who is now 23 and a pediatric nurse, says that Aaron taught her at an early age to be more patient and inclusive, accepting and non-judgemental.

Aaron's older brother Isaac shares similar sentiments, adding that Aaron has greatly strengthened his compassion. And Mike, Aaron's dad, emphasizes that Aaron has challenged him in ways he didn't expect, but also warns not to underestimate your child's ability to learn or enjoy the things you enjoy.

For example, Aaron loves swimming competitively, watching hockey and eating French fries just like his dad. The majority of children's genes come from their mom and dad. For Aaron, it is only the one chromosome that is extra.

Ella once said to me, "I wish other people could see Aaron as I see him." This is why it is so important for all people who work with children with disabilities – health care professionals, therapists, educators – to take the time to understand the actual reality of families. Often people have stereotypes of disabilities stuck in their head, just as I had when Aaron was first born. We all must confront our own ableism if we are to create inclusive environments where everybody belongs.

Aaron has taught me that different is not bad; it is just different. Much of my own suffering in life comes from pining for a different life. I had to move through acceptance to celebration of Aaron in my own time. Yes, some things are harder, but the important things require hard work. I've also discovered that I can do hard things.

Families need to know that they and their child can – and will – live a good and rich life. Professionals can help by sharing authentic stories of other families, reminding them to take care of themselves and connecting families up with each other.

But the most crucial thing that people can do when working with families of disabled children is to be aware of their own personal values about disability. It is their responsibility to do their research and check those values against the actual lived experience of families and children.

For it is love, patience and faith that will help guide a family's way. Health professionals – in particular – are in a unique position to help families begin their child's life as a celebration and not a tragedy.

Neck Deep in Health Care

~ a glimpse into the effect of cold and brusque appointments ~

All of the organization, the burden of uncertainty, of management, the coordination of care, the careful communication, has worn me down.
– Isabel Jordan

My treks to the doctor's office exploded when Aaron was diagnosed. Suddenly he and I were both immersed in hospitals, clinics, labs and waiting rooms. Oh, the waiting rooms I've seen.

First we had an appointment with the genetics clinic. They thought they saw a cataract in his eye. So then he got bounced to ophthalmology.

After ophthalmology (he had what they actually termed "gunk" in his eye, not a cataract), he was referred to cardiology for an echocardiogram and ECG to make sure he didn't have a hole in his heart. He did have a hole in his heart, but it was the regular kind that closed on its own, called a VSD or ventricular septal defect. Meeting with the pediatric cardiologist remains one of the strangest encounters I've ever had with a doctor.

First, her resident came in and thoroughly listened to our little baby's heart. Apparently he had a small murmur. There was no chit-chat, just two trembling parents, terrified our baby needed heart surgery and a doctor with a cold stethoscope. He left the room. We waited alone in the room for a while, not knowing what was next. Then the pediatric cardiologist swooped in. I remember she was wearing very expensive shoes. I see that noticing the calibre of a physician's dress and shoes became a recurring theme for me.

"There's a murmur so come back in a year," she said brusquely. She was a brusque one. She took up so much room in the clinic that Mike, Aaron and I all shrunk in her presence. "Does he need surgery?" I ventured. "No," she said dismissively, waving her hand. I'll never forget what happened next.

She turned her back to us and started dictating her clinic notes into a dictation machine. This was 2003, remember, before the fancy computer dictation devices that they have now. "Aaron Wadding-ham, with Down syndrome…" My husband and I glanced at each other. Was our appointment done? Was this our good-bye? Our cue to leave?

We gathered up Aaron and our things and crept out the door. That was that. While I'm used to a doctor writing a prescription to signal the end of the appointment, I'd never been dismissed by a doctor turning her back and talking into a device about our son, who was right there in the room. It was cold, odd and disheartening. I don't think that hospital folks truly understand how these experiences can deeply affect patients. For many staff, it is just routine. For us, it could be the worst day of our lives. Thankfully we never had to see her again. The hole in his heart closed on its own and that was that.

There were other appointments too: an extensive hearing test, a set of diagnostics to investigate his kidneys because he kept getting infections, the pulmonologist because he had sleep apnea, the ear, nose and throat (ENT) specialist who eventually took out his tonsils, the pediatric orthopedic surgeon because he was born with a dislocated knee, the pediatric dental surgeon who extracted some of his wonky teeth under anesthetic.

I remember bits from all these encounters. I remember how gentle the dental hygienist was with him in the dentist's office. How she explained what she was doing step by step. To this day he happily goes to the dentist and has none of the dental anxiety that I acquired as a child. The ENT doctor was from South Africa. In his wonderful accent, he explained to Aaron that he was looking for bunnies in his ears.

It was Dr. Darwish, his beloved pediatrician, who arranged all these referrals and appointments. One day she said to me, "He's a healthy boy with Down syndrome. He can go to a family physician now." I was conflicted by this: happy that his health stuff settled down, but sad we weren't going to see her anymore. A few months later, I found out why. Dr. Darwish was finding spots for all the kids in her practice because she had cancer and was dying at age 52.

The funeral home was so packed for her service that they had to put a video feed in the overflow room. At her funeral, there were many familiar faces of people with Down syndrome who had been cared for by her over the years. Her obituary asked for donations to the local Down syndrome society. Her life had touched so many children and families. Our tears flowed down the street that day.

Doctor in the Snazzy Dress

~ getting down to the level of the patient, no matter how small ~

We are guests in our patients' lives.

– Don Berwick

When Dr. Azza Darwish died, Aaron was only two, so we had to find another pediatrician. Thankfully Azza had trained many pediatric residents over the years. One of them was Dr. Mel Lewis, a former nurse who went to medical school and was mentored by Dr. Darwish. We were fortunate that Dr. Lewis (call me Mel, she said) had nurtured a love for patients with Down syndrome in her time with Azza and opened up her practice to accept many of her orphaned patients. She became Aaron's new pediatrician.

I have been thinking about how I built trust with Mel. I remember the first time meeting this wonderful doctor. She knocked on the clinic door, said hello, and immediately zoomed in on engaging Aaron. She charmed both of us with her approach, which was friendly, open and sincere. My first impression was: gosh, she's a snazzy dresser. My second impression was: wow, look at her sitting cross-legged on the clinic floor in her nice dress, chatting with my two-year-old boy. The great thing about pediatricians is that they love kids. I'm not sure the adult health world can always say the same thing about their patients.

Of course Aaron's pediatrician is technically proficient and clinically-competent. The first time he was hospitalized, he got crackerjack care from her. Her nurse coordinator also does a fabulous job of responding to questions from families, even when she's swamped with work, which has saved us (and the system) from many clinic and emergency room visits.

I think I trusted our pediatrician because she presented to me as a person first. She's a mom, too, and I know that she has three boys. I knew she was a nurse before she became a doctor, and we ran into her in our community – at the recreation centre, in the grocery store. I connected with her on a human level. She allowed me a glimpse into her own life as a mom, and this helped form the bond of trust with her. I have to confess: if I trust a health professional, I will do just about anything for them. I am very "compliant" (gosh, I hate that word) for people I trust. If I don't like you – I'm not very motivated to do as you say.

I think if you communicate that you care about me, I will work extra hard to care for myself. As a patient this is true, and the same applies as the mom of a patient, too.

So yes, I trusted Aaron's doctor. But this isn't blind trust – this is mutual trust, based on demonstrated caring and the gradual piecing together of a human relationship. And in today's world of informed patients, trust does need to be nurtured by clinicians, and by patients too. And that might start with sitting on the clinic floor in your snazzy dress.

Relearning How to be a Mother

~ pondering about changing my disabled child to fit into the world ⌒

First I wanted to change my child so he would fit in the world.
Then I wanted to change the world so they would accept my child.
Then I realized that I was the one who needed changing.

– Anonymous

The changing of my child so he would fit into the world is a strong push from professionals in the early years. First, I was given a book about babies with Down syndrome that listed everything that could possibly go wrong with my child and all the ways to fix it. I became obsessed with arranging therapists to come to our home to fix my baby. There was a regular parade of occupational therapists and physiotherapists sitting on the living room floor with our son. I'd have pages of photocopied sheets of paper with homework that I was to do with him between visits.

At first, I was keen, practicing picking up Cheerios with Aaron to perfect his pincher grasp for hours at a time. Then I got tired and Aaron did too. By this time, I was caring for four other children in my home at various times – the sum of our messy blended family –

Isaac and Ella and Mike's two sons, who were all under the age of 10 when Aaron was born.

In the early years, Aaron had a ton of appointments at the hospital for various specialists. The coordination of these medical appointments was in itself dizzying. I was also recovering from childbirth and deep in emotional grief too. I kept going because what choice did I have? I loved my baby and wanted the best for him. My husband had many mouths to feed and was back at work the day after Aaron's diagnosis. Once I had bundled up the other children and taken them to school, it was me and my little baby at home all day. I was both strung out with grief and terribly lonely, despite being surrounded by health professionals. If someone asked how I was doing, I'd cheerily say "Fine!" and that was that. Nobody ever dug any deeper and neither did I.

I know that the clinicians at the hospital had no idea what was going on for the seven of us at home, because nobody ever asked. Each specialty looked at Aaron as a separate body part. The ENT looked at his ears, nose and throat, the audiologist only looked at his ears, the cardiologist only listened to his heart. He was fractured into pieces and I was the only one who had his whole picture.

After a year, I became weary of the therapists' assigned homework. Soon I became a slacker, pulling out the homework sheets half an hour before the professionals came to my door to half-heartedly encourage Aaron to keep his tongue in his mouth or sit up unsupported. I went through the motions because this was what I was expected to do. The silent assumption was that we all needed to work hard to create the best baby with Down syndrome ever, or worse, to make our children appear as "normal" as possible.

I think there's a difference between supporting families and fixing them, but nobody ever asked my opinion. I was just another mom in a heavy workload – tired and weary, but putting on a happy face when the parade of professionals arrived at my front door. Mostly, I wish that someone had asked me how I was really doing. I learned to keep my "strong Mom" persona on for the health professionals who paraded through Aaron's life.

On the other hand, all children do benefit from early intervention. But how do we decide what interventions, and how much? I was most concerned about Aaron's speech, but that was the one professional who was not assigned to him. Nobody asked, what is important to you? The system was just focused on what they thought Aaron needed, not what mattered to our family. There was no flexibility there – he was seen as a Down syndrome diagnosis, not as a unique human being. It is a precarious balance between helping our children be their best and giving them space to flourish.

Are we over-fixing our children so they can fit into the world? Is this being done in the pursuit of making our children the best they can be? I have heard a number of young adults with disabilities say, "When my parents sent me to therapy, it gave the message to me that I was broken." I wonder now if it was me that was broken, not my son. What in the world did he have to be rehabilitated from?

I now know that I was the one who needed changing. I've only accepted my son through my own internal process of having a long look at my own misconceptions about disabled people. This is hard, humbling work. If I really do love all my children unconditionally, as I say I do, this means that love for Aaron is not conditional on erasing the third copy of his 21st chromosome. Aaron, I love you just the way you are.

You've Got a Friend in Me

an essay on how health professionals
can help families find peer support

When I think of that time now, I think of hands.

– Jennifer Graf Groneberg

All mothers need support. When I first became a mother 26 years ago, I had no sisters, I was a relatively young mom with distant parents, and none of my friends were having babies yet. I found groups of mom friends when my older two (typically developing) children were born. The other moms I met in my neighbourhood and at playgroups provided me with cheerleading and companionship I needed during a pivotal time in my life, as I adjusted to my new role of being a mother.

I have been preaching about the value of peer support for families who have children with disabilities for a long time. Parents inherently know that peer support is valuable. Professionals can be leery of such endeavours, citing risk and encroachment on their scope of practice or professional boundaries. But peer support is not just a "nice thing to do" – research shows that it helps parents gain confidence and hope in challenging situations.

Peer support looks different for everybody. Peer support must be delivered by peers, not professionals. With training and experience, this is one thing that families can do all by themselves. Yet families aren't going to stalk the hospital hallways looking for another baby with Down syndrome. We need help – from health professionals – to find each other. This is about having the option to contact another parent if we so desire. It is about choice.

All families and patients with an unexpected diagnosis need to be given the option to be connected up with their peers in the early days. This can be through Neonatal Intensive Care units (NICUs), on maternity units, in rehab facilities, via home care, in early intervention – anywhere families who have babies or children with unexpected news can be found.

> *When I think of that time now, I think of hands. Hands working for us, some belonging to people I've known for years...others were strangers to me – nurses whose names I could barely keep straight, social workers, doctors, neighbours I knew just by sight. Hands folded in prayer...hands dialing phone numbers as our news spread...wherever I went, it seemed I was never alone. I felt cradled, loved; led by so many that it became one, one love, one light, leading me home. –Jennifer Graf Groneberg[1]*

When Aaron was born with Down syndrome, I found myself utterly and painfully alone, sitting on the couch, holding my boy. I attempted a Mom and Baby Yoga class, but fled after one mom asked me that prenatal testing question. I tried a music class for moms and babies, but another mom's joke about "slow kids" hurt so much that I never went back.

> *One well-meaning nurse said to me, "You'll get used to it. You'll get thick skin." I didn't want thick skin. I wanted my dreams back. –Jennifer Graf Groneberg*

SUE ROBINS

I had to create, from scratch, a new dream for my son, my family, and me. I slowly found my new community of moms.

I'll never forget the first time I met a mom who had a three-year-old daughter with Down syndrome. Aaron must have been two months old. I was shaking with nerves when I arrived at her house.

She graciously welcomed us, and immediately asked if she could hold Aaron. Her face lit up as she held him, and she said, "Oooooh, this makes me want to have another baby." I thought she'd gone mad – my baby had Down syndrome. I thought, "Why in the world would you want that?"

This mom was three years into her journey with her daughter, and she was so much wiser than fragile, vulnerable me. Watching her daughter sit on the playroom floor and flip through board books gave me hope for the future that my son would one day read (and yes, today he does read). In her unabashed delight for my son, I knew that everything was going to be okay.

This other mom showed me how to love my boy, and most importantly in our world, how to accept him too. That's a lesson that is not taught by professionals. We can only learn that from each other, but we need opportunities to meet.

The key thing is that we often need professionals to help us find each other. It was our pediatrician, Dr. Darwish, who encouraged us to attend a Down syndrome support group meeting to connect with other parents. That simple encouragement was all we needed to start on our way. Peer support works – just give us the chance, and we will take it from there.

Finding other moms who had babies with Down syndrome is what saved me. Sixteen years ago, there were no mom's groups – but four moms with our tiny, flexible babies with almond eyes found each other. We would get together every month at each other's houses with our wee ones. Helga, Veronica and Karen were my saving grace. They knew what it was like to have an unexpected child with Down syndrome and we could talk to each other freely and without judgement.

Today Aaron is friends with these (now) teenagers, who he first met when he was five months old. He and Helga's son Vincent spend a glorious weekend each summer on their family boat – endlessly jumping off into the lake, tubing and engaging in rowdy burping contests. Aaron and Veronica's son Andrew regularly FaceTime each other. I can hear the two of them roaring with laughter on the iPad in Aaron's room. Aaron and Karen's daughter Gracie recently had a lovely lunch with one another. These friendships are essential for Aaron too.

Mothering any child is hard. We all need support, disability or not, and I wish our world was kinder to moms in general. I feel thankful for my trail of mom friends. Is peer support valuable? Hell yes. What is peer support, but caring for another human being? These women don't provide peer support to me. We are simply each other's friends.

Notes
1. Graf Groneberg, Jennifer, Roadmap to Holland, 2008.

I'm a Difficult Mom

∽ the story behind why patients and families become difficult ◡

We don't know "difficult families" but difficult situations are something we see plenty of – mainly caused by shrinking resources that neither family nor services have any control over.
– Marianne Selby-Boothroyd and Liz Wilson

I once got up in front of an audience of staff and physicians in a hospital and announced: *I am a difficult mom.* I added: *If your child was hospitalized, you'd be a difficult mom too.*

As with most of my talks, my intention was for the staff to see themselves reflected in my words. I asked them to think how they would respond if they had a concern when their loved one was in the hospital. I can't imagine that most health professionals would be meek and compliant family members.

I talked about the reasons why families can be challenging partners, which includes a list of significant factors: loss of control; fear; pain; grieving; information overload; feeling hopeless; cultural differences with staff, leading to assumptions and miscommunication; fear of negatively affecting their child's care if they speak up.

There are certain practical things that can make this worse. Lack of sleep. No coffee. Being hungry. Worry about other kids at home.

Concern about money and work. Compound that with stress about their beloved child-patient and you create a difficult situation, not a difficult family.

I gently suggested: *Please pause and always consider how families are feeling. You might not be able to put yourself in their shoes, but you may be able to move towards a kinder understanding of their perspective.*

Often anger can be misdirected – and sometimes it is not. People may indeed be angry at you! This is a great time for self-reflection, to think about why this may be, instead of dismissing and stereotyping them as "difficult families." Many families in the health system are deep in the throes of grief, and of course being stuck in anger is very common in grief. Perhaps something in their experience has triggered a traumatic response.

Patients can be reeling from a new diagnosis, in the purgatory of waiting for a diagnosis, grappling with a catastrophic incident or accident that has changed every aspect of their own lives, or (not so simply) be worn down by the system. Everything in health care feels like a wait, a struggle, a fight.

Ironically (or not), health care organizations do not make things easier for patients to access care, they make it more difficult. Say I am sick and I've been waiting for this appointment for six months. I sat in your waiting room for 55 minutes. The receptionist was rude to me. I got lost trying to find your clinic. Parking, when I finally found it, emptied out my wallet. I have to go pick up a kid from school soon. No wonder we can be crappy partners. We need you to help us work with you. Listening helps. Being open to our questions helps. Follow up helps. Being kind helps.

I said to my audience of staff and doctors: *There are many reasons patients and families are crappy partners. Instead of expecting us to come to the table just like you – well dressed, of decent income, well rested, educated, understanding the lingo and the system – why not recognize where we are at?*

I made it clear in this talk that I don't dismiss the real concern of patients being abusive towards staff. This is not okay. But there are many shades of anger – and I believe the best reaction when one is struggling with another human being is to step back and think: *Where is this person coming from?*

In a system that does its best to dehumanize people, taking the time to understand patients makes them human again.

Reframing Complaints

⟿ reconsidering the whole process of patient and family feedback ⟿

**It isn't about who is right, or who is smarter; it is about
what is in the best interest of that family member everyone
is trying to support. And this is where the two perspectives
together are greater than the sum of their parts.**

– Yona Lunsky

T he convoluted, cloaked patient complaint process is an example
of how most hospitals would like to bury complaints deep in the
earth. The only way things are going to improve is if organizations become more transparent and open to admitting they made a mistake.

I'd prefer to reframe complaints as constructive feedback.

Why not look at complaints as valuable feedback to inform health
care's quality improvement projects? If you openly collect the feedback data and identify themes – voilà! Change to the hospital can
occur based on what matters to the patients and families. This is
patient centred quality improvement.

This feedback can be related to care or service at the hospital, or
more broadly, at the organizational level. Take that valuable feedback

– which is gold – and apply it to improve things for next time around.

There's another, more insidious result of poor management of patient concerns. Many patients and families are worried about being labelled as difficult. So many moms have come to me and said, fearfully, "They think I'm a hysterical mom." I can't tell them, "No, that's not true" because this does happen.

I say, "It is your job to stand up for your child. You are doing the right thing. Keep going." The reluctance to speak up stems from a fear that doing so might affect their child's care or service. There is no a safe place to speak up. So they wait and things build and build and build until the whole thing explodes.

I think of a concern starting from a patient or family standing on the edge of a steep cliff with this boulder of an issue. Once the issue starts rolling down that mountain, it gains more and more momentum and power and it is really hard to stop it. Let's help patients and families when they are standing at the edge of the cliff, before things get out of control.

In my experiences meeting with families with escalated concerns, I learned this: 90% of the source of the concern was that people did not feel heard. Simply making the space for the listening helped. Of course, concerns are always complex – they involve wait times, and process problems too. But much of what families shared with me was feedback about how they were treated. They felt dismissed, ignored and labelled.

To create spaces where people feel safe to speak up, there has to be a recognition of the power imbalance between patients/families and health professionals. It is essential to shift from telling people what to do to listening and learning from people instead.

The philosophy of creating the listening space for concerns can be a challenging concept for those who are used to "fixing" problems. Some problems are not to be fixed. They are to be listened to.

There are often practical solutions that come with concerns – getting off wait lists, having stern conversations with rude staff – which of course need to be addressed. The most important piece is to try to prevent concerns from happening. If this isn't possible, the next piece is how concerns are handled. Are they ignored, buried, dismissed? The angriest of all patients will say yes, this is what health organizations do.

Delaying response to a concern makes it even worse, and layers yet another concern on top of the original one: lack of responsiveness. Then there are two concerns, not just one. Vow to have a standard response time to patient and family concerns. Pick up the phone. Arrange an in-person meeting. Any response can help de-escalate the situation and prevent further misunderstandings.

In the pediatric world, families who have experienced adverse events have the most valuable of all feedback to share. It is in fact an honour for health organizations to have patients approach them with their stories. The wisdom generated from when things go wrong is very powerful. Patients and families are driven to influence change so the event doesn't happen to anybody else. This gives some meaning to often traumatic and sad situations. Some of the best patient council members are those who found their way to the boardroom table through a concern or an adverse event. Do not be afraid of these patients and families – they can help you with your work.

But in order to be open to learning from concerns, one must learn humility. Hospital culture must allow for mistakes, make them visible and transparent, and support their staff to respond to errors in a respectful way.

Don't push people away and squash their voices. That makes it worse. Say yes instead of no as much as possible. Say you are sorry this has happened. This does not assign blame to you, it merely expressed regret for something that has happened. The power of apology is strong. Listen. Don't interrupt.

Pause and think – how would I feel if it was me?

A final point: patients or families offering up feedback can help you in your work. From experience, I know best how to explain blood draws to Aaron or how to comfort him when he's upset. Families can help professionals if only we work together as a team, for we each have our own unique expertise to bring to the bedside. Remembering that we are all on the same team will only benefit the patient in the end.

The Hospital World According to Aaron

~ on not forgetting the person who had the experience ⌒

I AM NOT DEAD!

– Aaron

Aaron had day surgery at our children's hospital when he was 11 years old. In an effort not to be a 'secret shopper', I try to take my family centred care hat off when I'm in the hospital with my boy. I focus on him as opposed to critiquing every single interaction.

My youngest son has had four surgeries in his life, and this was the first time I did not push the pre-sedation request. Aaron was relaxed and joking with the nurses, so I thought, "Let's just see what happens if he doesn't get sedation before he goes into the operating room." I warned him there would be lots of people and bright lights in the OR, and he was perfectly fine (I now wonder if the pre-sedation request was more for me: Mom needs sedation). It is fortunate that our hospital has parental presence at induction, which means I was able to go into the OR with him until he was asleep. I teared up a bit when he was put under, as I always do – and the kind anesthetist said to me, "We will take good care of him." And that they did.

93

Afterwards, I reflected on Aaron's own experience as a patient. He was annoyed that he had to wear a dress. Apparently, the hospital switched to gowns for kids and don't use pajamas any more. He had to wear a mask because he had a cough. Sensory-wise, that was not great – it was scratchy and bothered him and he kept taking it off.

Despite the fact that we explained the going to sleep part, the first thing he shouted when he woke up after surgery was, "I AM NOT DEAD!" I'm horrified he thought he might have died – I am constantly in awe of how this kid's mind works. I harkened back to earlier in the year when we had to put our beloved chocolate lab "to sleep" and realized I needed to adjust my own explanations and avoid euphemisms. In Aaron's mind, the dog died after he was put to sleep, so why shouldn't he? Oy. Point well taken.

The day surgery unit was busy and unfortunately, some of the kids didn't wake up well after surgery, so there was a fair bit of crying and screaming. There was also a considerable amount of construction noise – hammering and drilling. "I don't like hospitals," Aaron told me. I asked why.

"I don't like these screaming kids. It is too noisy here," he said. I realized that a less open physical space would have worked better for him, a boy with auditory sensory issues. He wouldn't even consider the Popsicle the nurses offered him after surgery. He said, "The food here is disgusting," drawing upon his (accurate) memory as a hospital inpatient.

"I want to go home," he concluded. Ask him about his own patient experience, and this is what you get – he is a fountain of truth.

I'm grateful for his uneventful experience. I'm also thankful for the folks at the hospital who cared for him: the clerk at reception, the practical nurses, the recovery room nurses, the porters, the surgeon, the OR nurses and the anesthetist. They all had smiles on their faces, spoke to Aaron directly and did their jobs competently.

This story is a gentle reminder that all surgery is a big deal to families and kids, even if it is considered "minor" to the professionals. I feel fortunate that Aaron's experience included such caring health professionals, and he went home safe and sound.

What is most interesting about this brief time in the hospital is Aaron's perception of it. For a child with Down syndrome and an identified intellectual disability, he communicated well about his own patient experience. It reminded me that none of us should speak up on his behalf, for he is quite capable of speaking up for himself.

This chapter is adapted from an essay originally published in the Journal of Paediatrics and Child Health, September 20, 2016.

SUE ROBINS

He Isn't a
Beeping Machine

∽ seeing the patient as a person first ⌒

...providing treatment should not be equated to offering care.
– Arthur Frank

I believe deeply in my heart that most people are drawn to health
professions with an initial passion to help others. This means
they care about others and want to make the world a better place.
This is a noble reason to choose a profession. Alas, once in practice, compassionate behaviour can begin to erode. I remember all
the kindnesses, and all the small cruelties too. The call bell never
answered when I needed help to go to the washroom. The refusal to
allow my husband into the room while I was getting an IV started.
The questions about Aaron directed at me when he was standing
right there.

There are all sorts of named excuses for this: no time, workload,
focus on technology and a preoccupation with tasks and to-do lists.
I don't think practitioners intend to forget their initial passion.
Simple reminders about what makes a difference for patients can
rekindle compassion in staff, and those reminders can come though

sharing patient stories about what matters to them.

My son was hospitalized for pneumonia twice, once when he was six years and again when he was 12. He was hooked to monitors that beeped and buzzed all day long – when his oxygen saturation fell, when his IV needed changing. All you could see in that big hospital bed was his little head popping out on the pillow. He lay there, sick and sad, too weak to move except for turning his eyes when someone came into the room.

It saddened me the number of times someone would burst into his room to adjust one of the beeping machines hooked up to him and yet not say a word to him. There was no acknowledgement that there was a little boy laying there, who had nothing to do except to watch the comings and goings of people in his space. Staff (who, nurses? Others? I don't know since they didn't introduce themselves) would rush in, rehang an IV bag and leave, not even looking at his little face peeking out from the scratchy bed linens. He searched their face, desperate for some eye contact or a hello that never came. It was as if this was a machine that happened to have a little boy connected to it, not a sick little boy attached to a machine.

For some staff, Aaron was an afterthought. They appeared rushed and frazzled, yes, but the 30 seconds spent adjusting the machine was spent in total silence. Would it have taken longer to say, "Hi Aaron! Good to see you! I'm your nurse, Dan, remember? Your machine is beeping and I'm here to fix it," while he was performing the task? No. No, it would not have added to that 30 seconds. The only thing it would have added was some humanity to an interaction with a sick little boy in a big hospital bed.

I remember those who demonstrated kindness. A knock on the door, a question that afforded choice: Is it okay if I come in? Perhaps there could be an introduction, a smile, some gentle conversation about the weather outside today and some explanation about why the machine was beeping. This could all be done while tackling the task at hand. This bedside manner does not take extra time. A return to the old-fashioned notion of bedside manner is exactly what's needed in today's efficiency-obsessed world of health care.

Handing Over our Kids

~ explaining the fear families feel when their kids are sick ~

**The sight of my son – stone-still on the OR table, deathly rigid –
completely unhinged my confidence that "everything would be okay."**
– Danielle Ofri

Physician and mom Danielle Ofri wrote an article in Slate about
being a mom who happens to have an MD and PhD – who faces
that mom-fear when her young son goes in for surgery.[1]

Danielle's words felt eerily familiar. I've always said there's nothing
worse than waiting for your child to come out of surgery. The good-
bye said in the OR feels awful. In that, it might be good-bye; I might
never see you again. Because things can go wrong in surgery: kids can
be allergic to anesthetic, or there's trouble intubating, or they can
have an incident in the OR, like a stroke. These things do happen.

Health professionals can help us parents manage that clammy,
stomach-churning fear.

Having parental presence at induction helps with anxiety. Instead
of handing a screaming kid over to a stranger, we go to the OR with
our children, and stay with them until they are asleep. While it is

disconcerting to see them knocked out, as mom Dr. Ofri says, it is calming to meet the OR staff, and know that our babies are well taken care of. Since my son has a cognitive disability, having sedation for him before going to the OR when he was younger helped with his anxiety level, too. He was fairly out of it when we reached the operating room, which was a terrifying place for a kid with sensory issues with shiny sharp instruments and very bright lights. OR staff can help us by introducing themselves, and explaining what their role is and what's going to happen next. This puts our kids' fears at ease too.

And the warm blankets! I think fondly of any warm blanket brought by a nurse or a porter to cover Aaron up as he is wheeled to the OR. Long live the warm blankets.

On an organizational level, hospitals can install systems that allow us to track our kids – to know when they are in the OR, and when they move to recovery. They can give us pagers to alert us when we can see our children. They can ensure there are private spaces for us to talk to the physician after surgery. They can have policies about parental presence both at induction and in the recovery room.

Danielle sums up the whole unthinkable situation well:

> My heart ached for parents whose children are truly ill, for the frightening bargain of uncertainty they must make as they entrust their children to the medical system.

Handing over your sick or frightened child to a complete stranger is what happens in pediatric health care all the time. Thankfully, we've moved beyond visiting hours in hospitals that allowed parents to only see children for a few hours every day. Children need their families and families need their children.

Notes

1. Ofri, Danielle, My Leap of Faith in Medicine, September 22, 2013, Slate.com. http://www.slate.com/articles/health_and_science/medical_examiner/2013/09/fear_of_medical_procedures_doctors_need_to_acknowledge_emotions.html

Work is Work is Work

∽ my foray into a career as a family advocate ∾

**The market wouldn't survive if it wasn't able to
survive on the backbone of unpaid work.**

– *Marilyn Waring*

A medical student once asked me, "Did having a child with a disability affect you financially?" Why yes, yes it did. After Aaron was born, I did not return to my full-time job with the Ministry of Health. Aaron had many hospital appointments and home visits with early intervention staff and therapists. The scheduling of all these appointments was a part-time job. I was the coordinator of everything. Daycare spots for a disabled kid were hard to secure and we didn't have the money to hire a nanny. I left the traditional workforce and fell into freelance writing.

Being a freelancer is not necessarily a bad thing, but it still bugs me that I didn't have a choice in the matter. Workplaces are notoriously not family-friendly, particularly for caregivers. Here I must mention my privilege. My husband was a full-time IT consultant when Aaron was born. We could afford to live on his one income while I scratched around for freelance writing gigs. I began writing health features for a food magazine, which morphed into writing for a health region and then into feature writing for health regulatory body magazines. It took time to build a reputation, but I did it during Aaron's naps, one article at a time.

Yes, we lost considerable income and security when I left my cushy full-time position. But in that loss there is a gain. I suddenly had freedom that comes with freelancing – freedom to set my own hours, to arrange my schedule, to work when it was best for my family. That in itself was a gift. I walked away from the full-time cubicle job, never to return. Aaron granted me this. As with many things about having a child with a disability, this new work set-up was different but not bad. It was just different. Different was becoming a running theme in my life.

When Aaron was two, he attended a speech class at a local rehabilitation hospital. A social worker facilitated a mom's support group while Aaron was in class. There I met other moms, which is always a godsend, and I was asked if I wanted to join the new family council at the hospital. This was 2005. Naïve me said, sure! I have some ideas about how to make the speech program better! I did not realize that I was unwittingly on the forefront of the family council movement that was ramping up in the early 2000s in Canada.

I am a big mouth and a keener so soon I started chairing a national group of family councils in Canada. This, too, was unpaid work. I did it because I believed that including the family voice could only improve the health system. Patient and family centred care was starting to be a thing in children's health.

As many mothers do, I carefully pieced together paid and unpaid work. My unpaid work included looking after my little baby, two kids and two stepchildren. I was in the "I'm going to save the world" phase of having a child with a disability, so I volunteered like mad. I had not slowed down enough to realize the only person I could really save was myself.

Then a wonderful thing happened. The local acute care children's hospital knew of my volunteer work with councils. There was a champion there, a director who had a brother with Down syndrome. We connected at conferences and in the hallways. She invited me to speak to the leadership team at the hospital to pitch the idea of starting a family council there.

I nervously dug up my old business suit and walked into a room of intimidating women, all senior leaders at the hospital. With my heart beating hard, I gave my most heartfelt speech about the value of family councils to guide improvements at the hospital. My director friend ushered me out afterwards and whispered in my ear at the elevator, "I'll send over a contract for you next week."

I became one of those lucky people who get paid to do what they love. I became a family centred care consultant, a job which I was previously doing for free. Now I was getting paid. This was a 60–hours-a-month position. I told them I did not want a desk at the hospital. Instead I came in for meetings but mostly spent my time in the community, connecting with families at coffee shops and in their homes. These types of jobs – now called patient engagement positions – are really outreach positions. You go to where the people are. You don't sit in your office and expect them to come to you.

Family engagement is what moved our family out to the west coast of Canada, when I took a part-time position as the family engagement advisor at a pediatric rehabilitation hospital. There I learned a valuable lesson: staff need to be engaged so that patients and families are engaged. Staff morale affects patient care. Staff and patients are so intertwined that there's no unwinding them. What happens to one affects the other because health care is about relationships between human beings.

Almost two years in, I had to take a leave from my family engagement advisor job to care for my own son, who was teetering on adolescence. I requested a more flexible work schedule, but I was denied. So I resigned, distraught that what I thought was my life's work in children's hospitals was over after only 10 years.

Three days after my last day of work, I went to my family physician's office, concerned about a lump I found in my left breast.

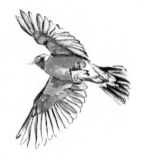

The Cancer

When One
Door Closes

∿ the fragility and unexpectedness of life ∽

See when it starts to fall apart
Man, it really falls apart.

– Tragically Hip

My grief about the loss of my job and my associated identity
ran deep. Many people informed me, "When one door clos-
es, another one opens." I waited for the other door to open.

My one silver lining about being unemployed was that I suddenly
had newfound time on my hands. I had five precious hours each day
while my son was at school. I had officially run out of excuses not to
write a book.

As a writer, I had my essays published in health journals and
newspapers. A story about my eldest son was published in the Sunday edition of *The New York Times*. This is awesome, but once you see
yourself in print in *The Times*, it feels like you've reached some sort
of pinnacle and it is all downhill from there. It took me some time to
recover from this feeling and realize that there can be other peaks to
climb too. One of those mountaintops is a book.

I started my book project and titled it *Ducks in a Row*. Its purpose was to share stories of patient engagement based on years as a paid and unpaid family advisor in children's health care. I had learned a lot about what was meaningful engagement in an organization and what was merely tokenism.

I started madly writing and researching patient and family centred engagement at our local university. Home alone, I struggled with motivation to keep me writing every day. I was the expert in doing everything but work – meeting friends for lunch, shopping, errand running and Twitter surfing.

I still managed to cough up 70,000 words. I was done my first draft and was preparing yet procrastinating on doing a first edit and polishing sample chapters to start shopping for a publisher. Everything was going according to plan for a few idyllic weeks. I was blissfully unaware that I was actually teetering on the edge of a cliff on my way up the mountaintop.

One night my husband and I were lying in bed giggling along with the Netflix show *Unbreakable Kimmy Schmidt*. I stretched and placed my hand over the left side of my chest, near where my heart was. It was then I felt something I had not felt before.

I said nothing to my husband and shrugged it off. The next day I Googled "lump in breast", and was met with a barrage of search results. I scanned them all and decided to choose the result I wanted. It was the one that said, "A lump in your breast is likely benign and it may be cyclical. Monitor it for a month to see if it goes away." So that's what I did.

A month later, it had not gone away. It was there, all ominous, more of a ridge than a lump. Even though I didn't want to know what it was, I broke down and made an appointment with my family doctor.

This first appointment was the beginning of a barrage of appointments over the next three months, each marching eerily towards a diagnosis.

In the meantime, there was the book. Since denial is an effective method of pain control, I continued writing *Ducks in a Row* cloaked by deep denial in between medical appointments.

As time crept on, the notion that I might have breast cancer was never far from my thoughts. Whenever the c word crept in, I shoved it deep in the back of my brain. The more diagnostic appointments I attended, the more cancer became my constant companion. A cold wash of fear settled in my belly, unrelenting, 24 hours a day.

I became unable to think. Any intellect that I may have possessed vanished from my body. I struggled to continue cheerily writing a book about patient engagement when I was neck-deep in an impending health crisis.

This was the beginning of my great humbling. I spent my days in early 2017 scattered and immersed in terror, merely existing to wait for the next phone call or medical appointment that brought me closer to my inevitable day of diagnosis.

I started a rambling personal journal called *Grace Period* that was anything but graceful. At first, it was mostly a chronological telling of my various medical appointments. At this point, I become obsessed with the appointments and phone calls and jumped every time my phone rang.

December 11, 2016

Wait for the radiologist to fax my doctor the report.

Thursday December 14 morning – my doctor calls to say she's sending a referral to the women's hospital. They should call me right away to set up an appointment in the next week to 10 days.

Nobody calls me. I call my doctor's office Thursday. Then Friday. Get the number for the Breast Health Clinic. I leave a message there Friday at

12:30 pm.

What else can I do but wait.

My writing days faded down to a couple of hours a week until a few weeks later, when progress on my book became hopelessly stuck in a snowdrift of cancer anxiety.

I do not know if I would have been more okay if I'd had a regular job to go to every day. Maybe a job would have served as a distraction? This was not my reality. Instead I was at home by myself, surrounded by my dark thoughts. I told nobody about this breast cancer scare, except for my husband.

On one hand, I feared crying wolf and unsettling everybody if my testing came back negative. On the other hand, I desperately needed someone to talk to, but there was nobody. My husband didn't want to talk about it and who can blame him? All the health professionals said, "Oh, don't worry. It is probably nothing."

But I did worry. And it wasn't probably nothing.

There is value in having someone – anyone – to talk to while one is in the middle of the diagnostic odyssey for cancer. A patient navigator? A cancer peer support person? A social worker? I don't know who I needed to talk to, but I do know that great emotional harm was inflicted on me while I waited for the results to come back. It would have been a relief to talk to someone, even for a few minutes, about the fear and desperation that I was experiencing. It would have been reassuring to know what I was feeling was normal. It is normal to feel panic underscored by fear if you think you might have cancer.

One door had closed for me and another one slowly creaked open. Behind that open door was neither my book nor some great work opportunity. When the door to my job closed, behind the next door that opened was cancer.

My Own Private Purgatory

⌣ the pain caused by the process to get a cancer diagnosis ⌢

We need to stop just pulling people out of the river.
We need to go upstream and find out why they are falling in.
– Desmond Tutu

The time between my first mammogram and diagnosis took three excruciating months. I have had many worst times of my life and this was one of them. I was suspended for three months in an aura of numbness. No wonder the work of writing a book fell by the wayside.

My travels through diagnostics started out well, beginning with my family physician listening to me as I described a ridge in my breast that she couldn't detect.

She said, "If you are worried about it, I'll send you for a mammogram." She could have dismissed me or told me I was perimenopausal and the ridge was normal, but she detected the worry in my voice and arranged the mammogram. I was 48 years old and had never had a mammogram. Our province recommends mammograms at age 50. I hate to think of how big my tumour would have grown in two years if my doctor hadn't listened to my concern.

It was at the diagnostic imaging place that things started to go downhill. There were many women there for mammograms and fear hanging in the air. I went in for the boob squishing and was told to sit back in the waiting room.

It was in an open room surrounded by other scared women that I was told there were abnormalities in my mammogram.

"The radiologist says you need an ultrasound. We could do it right now, but your doctor didn't check ultrasound on the requisition so you have to go back to see her to get a new requisition form," I was told.

At that time I should have spoken up and insisted on getting the ultrasound done right then and there. Instead I just smiled and nodded, in a weird sort of shock. This was the beginning of the delay of my diagnosis.

I don't know why the radiologist was unable to make an exception and grant me an ultrasound right then and there. I never met this person, as he or she sent the technician out to do the work of talking to patients. I think the radiologist must have had an inkling that a suspicious mammogram would cause a patient anxiety. Instead he or she decided to exacerbate that anxiety by making me book an appointment with my family physician, go see her, get another requisition and then book another appointment for the ultrasound. This process took another three weeks.

In my head, I was thinking that the delay was inconvenient but no big deal because I didn't have cancer, right? But here's the thing. The radiologist knew that there was a possibility that I could have cancer. This person wasn't in denial. They chose to delay my diagnosis because of a missed checkmark on a piece of paper. This seems especially cruel to me.

I arrived back at the imaging place three weeks later with the correct form in hand. The ultrasound took forever. I had two ultrasounds by two different technicians, but I don't know why I had two because they never told me. It seemed they needed to validate each other's results? I was there for a long time. Each minute seemed like I was inching towards my doom. This time I was again in an open waiting area, surrounded by a new set of scared women, when I was informed I'd need more diagnostic tests – this time a biopsy. I had my head down and didn't look at anybody. You poor sucker, they were probably thinking. Why can't this significant and private health information be disclosed in a private space?

"Go to the front desk and book the biopsy," I was told.

Obediently I got dressed and went to the front desk. By now I felt as if I was floating over my body, just as when Aaron was diagnosed with Down syndrome.

I saw myself talking to the receptionist. She says she can get me in for a biopsy in three days. A biopsy is bad news, but getting in quickly for a biopsy is good news. I'm freaked out inside but also grateful.

It was early December, a month after I initially saw my family doctor. I felt a need to mention to the receptionist that I have a bleeding disorder. I have a mild version of Von Willebrand Disease, which is a blood clotting disorder. This means that I take a long time to stop bleeding. Breast biopsies can evoke bleeding.

"I will go check with the (invisible) radiologist about that," said the receptionist and she disappeared. I was in a cold sweat in the main reception desk, and leaned heavily on the counter. I wished my husband was with me. I didn't anticipate that this appointment would go south. I shouldn't have mentioned my stupid bleeding disorder. This caused me great trouble.

The receptionist came back. "You can't get your biopsy done here on Friday," she informed me. The lady is pleasant enough, but firm. She must have sensed I might start begging her if I saw a crack in her demeanor.

"You have to go to a hospital and get it done." I have no idea how to do that. They won't help me at the diagnostic imaging place. I have to go back to my family physician (again) and be referred.

This takes a few more days. I visited my doctor to get the refer-ral. I'm rushing about, trying to get my Christmas shopping done, thinking irrationally that I might die before Christmas. Santa still has to come for my kids.

Life continued to swirl around me. Life doesn't care that I'm wait-ing to be called for a breast biopsy.

My Great Humbling

∽ the agony of waiting for appointments ⌒

The waiting is the hardest part.

– Tom Petty

On January 31, almost three months after my first visit with my doctor, I was scheduled for two biopsies at the local women's hospital. This was after an almost Abbott and Costello-like bumbling of the health care system that caused me an extra two months of waiting. It is difficult to describe how awful the waiting really is. It felt as if my brain was wading through fast-drying cement. I could only think fragments of thoughts at a time, interrupted by the words: cancer, cancer, cancer. I was barely functional. My days were random chaos, flitting from errand to errand in a desperate attempt to avoid my cancerous self.

At home, my dear husband, the eternal optimist, had convinced himself that my masses were benign, in the same way that I knew deep inside they were malignant. We didn't talk about the biopsies much, except in terms of logistics. Being unable to care for Aaron was one of my first and biggest fears about having cancer. I was frantic to find people to look after him. Thankfully, Mike's sister Jacqui stepped up for us. That was one worry off my long list of worries.

The biopsies did not go well. Mike was told I'd be in the procedure room for two hours. He obediently sat in the waiting room. I ended up being gone for four hours. Three hours in, sitting alone in the empty room, Mike figured out himself that something must be terribly wrong.

Inside the room, things ran over so long that I remember the mammogram technician calling her own doctor's office to reschedule her medical appointment so she could remain at work. They spent four hours alternating between squishing my breast in a mammogram machine, poking needles in my boob and using an archaic-looking device to extract eight pieces of my tissue from my body. I wasn't sedated and was wide awake for the entire experience. Thinking back, this was the first of many traumas that were inflicted on me in procedure rooms.

Towards the end of the appointment, I asked the radiologist, "Can you tell me anything at all?" She hesitated and said, "Well, you will have to have surgery, no matter what the pathology says." It was then I knew: one does not have surgery for a benign mass.

Three hours in, I pleaded, "Can someone go talk to my husband? He's been waiting this whole time." They wheeled me out so I could speak to him myself. He appeared in the hall, his brow furrowed and his face pale. "I'm almost done," I said. "They just have to bandage me up." He nodded sadly. I closed my eyes and shook my head.

Six days later, my family doctor's office called. "Dr. B would like to see you today," said the receptionist. She might as well have said, "I'm calling to tell you that you have breast cancer." It had snowed that day, a rare occurrence on the West Coast. We lived on top of a mountain and I knew it would take at least at hour to travel down to the medical clinic. "Just have her call me," I said. Then I phoned Mike and told him to come home right away.

At 4 p.m., my doctor called. Mike and I were sitting on our red couch, my cell phone on speaker. Aaron was set up in his bedroom, playing video games.

"Just tell me what's on the pathology report," I said, eager to forgo chitchat and get to the point. "You have a form of breast cancer," my young doctor said. She was just a year out of medical school and her voice was shaking. She read me the results of my report and informed me that my next step was to see a surgeon. "I hate doing this," she confessed later in the conversation. It was only then that I broke down and cried.

The diagnosis was not a surprise to me. I had been living with the "ridge" for four months now. The ridge kept me constant company. I carried it around all day long and then felt it at night as I lay in bed watching Netflix shows. We had gravitated to watching comedians like Dave Chappelle in a desperate attempt to keep things light so we could fall asleep at night. The biopsy appointment that ran into double overtime was a tell, as were the radiologist's ominous words. I knew I had breast cancer and it was simply confirmed by my doctor's call.

My husband, who had been living in sweet optimism before the call, was stunned at the news. His face immediately turned a shade of ash gray. There it was. His wife had breast cancer.

It was at that exact moment, at 4:06 p.m. on Monday, February 6, 2017, that I officially transformed from being a caregiver into being a patient.

Affronts to My Human Body

～ how the loss of dignity makes suffering worse ～

Out of suffering have emerged the strongest souls;
the most massive characters are seamed with scars.
– Edwin Hubbell Chapin

Pain and suffering cannot be totally eradicated in the cancer world. But I believe pain and subsequent suffering can certainly be mitigated by those who work in diagnostics and oncology.

Ignoring suffering only adds to the suffering. I think the lack of pain control measures during my various forays into cancer treatment – starting with the breast biopsy – increased my unnecessary suffering.

Breast biopsies are a strange combination of boob squishing, needle poking and tissue extraction. It is as awful as it sounds. I badly needed sedation for my biopsy, but none was offered.

Thankfully I popped my own anti-anxiety pill before the appointment. Sadly, after about an hour, my pill wore off and I still had three hours of biopsying to go.

The worst part of the biopsy was when they extracted the tissue from my breast with this weird box that contained a large bore needle that dug deep into my chest. My advice would be for all folks who are being biopsied: don't look down. I looked down to see a little box covered with my own blood. If I hadn't been lying down at that point, I would have hit the floor.

God help us all, including those who inflict the pain. No wonder health professionals experience their own suffering. My saving grace during the biopsy was the mammogram technologist, who kept stroking my hair during the procedure. This tender gesture is what got me through.

A few weeks later, after my eventual breast cancer diagnosis, it was the day of my partial mastectomy surgery. I was told to come to one hospital at 6:30 a.m. to get dye injected and then drive to another hospital across the city for my surgery.

Mike and I dutifully arrived at the first hospital at my appointed time, 6:30 a.m. I presented to the reception desk and the receptionist looked up at me and said sharply, "We don't open until 6:45 – take a number and sit down."

So many times patients are told to arrive 15 minutes early to their appointments. Listen, I am motivated to arrive on time if I possibly can for my cancer surgery. Why, oh why, would a hospital's process demand that I get there at 6:30 a.m. before it is even opened?

Like I was ordering deli meat, I took a number (I was Number 51) and sat down in the crowded, dirty waiting room. Posters were tacked up slightly askew on the walls and the fear was palpable in that little windowless room. We were mostly women waiting for breast cancer surgery – some alone, some, like me, lucky enough to have a partner by their side.

"Number 51," they eventually called. Mike and I stood up and followed the technician into the treatment room. I know they knew my name; being referred to as a number set an uncomfortable tone for the rest of the day.

I was unsure what to expect, but when I, as a layperson, think of an injection, I think of a needle in my arm. Nobody told me that the dye would be injected directly into my nipple.

The technician instructed me to take off my shirt and lay on the table. Take off my shirt? For a needle? I saw the horror spread across my husband's face. It dawned on both of us that I was about to get a needle in my breast. I didn't even realize the dye was being injected directly into my nipple until I felt the sharp sting of the needle.

Before I could protest, it was over and they were calling in the next poor patient. (As an aside: what a job to have, injecting dye in women's nipples all day long). The dye was apparently blue, because I had a blue nipple for months afterwards to remind me of this trauma.

This was not a good start to the day of my surgery.

My husband then drove me to the second hospital for my surgery.

I briefly thought to myself, "What if I wasn't a privileged person and I didn't have a car? Or I didn't have a husband to drive me? Would I have to take a bus by myself?" These seem like important questions for those in power to answer but I was too caught up in myself to consider changing the system at the moment.

At the second hospital, I was told to come in to the day ward. My husband remained in the waiting room. In a curtained pod, the nurse assembled the equipment to begin an IV.

"Can my husband come in now? I need him to hold my hand while the IV is started," I asked meekly, a confession of my needle fear.

"No," she said, not making eye contact with me. "He can come in after."

I shrunk back into my stretcher, feeling like a baby, afraid to make a fuss, hot tears forming in my eyes. The IV poke hurt, as did the tourniquet, and I had nobody to hold my hand.

I was wheeled down to radiology for the fine wire insertion in two spots in my left breast. I had no concept of what this meant.

The fine wire insertion involves inserting needles into my poor breast when it is squashed in a mammogram machine. It is the most horrific procedure I've endured in health care. This includes one time when it took seven tries to start an IV on the top of my foot. I was fully awake and already freaked out by impending surgery to cut out part of my breast. Plus, I had just found out I had cancer. I was not in a good emotional state.

The technician arranged me in the mammogram machine and the radiologist stuck me with needles. Then the radiologist inserted two wires in my breast. I was having trouble breathing and my big mistake was to look down. (Again, don't look down. Never look down). There were two long grey wires sticking out of my breast. I knew then I was about to faint. I was sweating, my head was ringing and I felt as if I was underwater.

I spoke up quietly, "Um, I'm sorry (sorry for what?) but I think I'm going to pass out."

This got their attention and I was allowed to have a rest before they continued on. The technician brought me rubbing alcohol which smelled just terrible. I felt like I needed something nice smelling instead, like lavender, along with a shot of morphine.

They informed me that fainting is common. Common! Why don't they do anything to alleviate it then? I was about to pass out from trauma and pain. How can this be okay, especially in a place where they were supposed to heal me?

I was even more fearful by the time I was brought back to the holding area to wait for surgery. I still can't believe they inflict this type of horror on women without any offer of medication. Thankfully my husband was finally allowed in and my daughter was there too so I felt some comfort from their presence.

It was starting to dawn on me how diagnostic imaging and procedures offer up all sorts of untold horrors in health care. I thought to myself before I was wheeled into surgery, "I can't go on. I must go on."

I had counselled my husband to ask the surgeon to speak with him afterwards so Mike could find out how my surgery went. "Okay," he said, strong, assertive and protective.

The conversation between the surgeon and Mike went like this:

Mike: "Can you come and tell me how it goes after Sue's surgery?"

Surgeon (laughs), "Oh no, I'm too busy to do that. There's a follow-up appointment in a couple of weeks." Two more long weeks of waiting.

I was knocked out for surgery and woke up again, groggy, with a bandage over my breast and under my arm. Back in the day ward afterwards, the nurse was eager to get me up and walking so they could discharge me. I was in a hospital gown that was flapping open at the back. Thankfully my daughter was by my side.

"Can she have a robe?" she asked, helping me out of bed.

"No, just tie up the gown," the nurse responded. No? I was cold and shivering and I had no clothes under the thin fabric gown. My daughter shook her head at the nurse, went to the supply cart, dug around for a robe and gently placed it around my shoulders. My girl walked with me, pushing my IV pole while I shuffled to the washroom.

This was a missed opportunity for simple kindness. What is particularly disturbing to me is that I know to ask for what I need. My family is not afraid to speak up. But we were all dismissed, disregarded and not listened to in the smallest but most significant ways.

I saw many people in the waiting room – what of the woman who was alone? Or the older lady who didn't speak English? Or the woman there for a double mastectomy, her sad husband by her side?

I am very fortunate that my dear daughter stayed with me for ten days after my surgery to be my caregiver. She distracted me, kept me company, fed me rice pudding, looked after her little brother, drove me around and tended to my dressings.

Before she left, she gave me a list of Ella Rules to consider. Rule number ten said: *Ignore stupid things – let yourself be upset but then let yourself move past it.* This is sage advice from a 20-year-old who has always been wise beyond her years.

As Ella advised, I endeavored to either politely respond to or shake off negative experiences. For my own mental health, I couldn't stew in this darkness while I waited for my cancer treatment to begin. I needed to stay in the moment and look for the light.

Where is
My Mama Bear?

~ the difference between being a caregiver and being a patient ~

**Find a bit of beauty in the world today. Share it. If you can't find it,
create it. Some days this may be hard to do. Persevere.**
– Lisa Bonchek Adams

While the term patient and family centred care lumps together both the patient and the family, I can now tell you
that the experiences are quite different. In my family, I was used to
looking after the patient/my son.

My job was to be a mama bear and I took this role very seriously.
I could hide behind my son in the role of mother to shield myself
from direct personal pain. Most of the job of being a mama bear is
being outraged – at systems, at society, at injustices, at uncaring professionals. Outrage is an all-consuming emotion that does a pretty
good job of blocking vulnerability. Mama bears aren't vulnerable!
They are fiercely protective and get easily angered if there is a whiff
that their child is threatened.

There's nowhere to hide when you have cancer. Cancer is deeply personal. There's also nobody to hide behind when you have

cancer. It strips you down to your own treacherous cells that have turned on you. It snatches away your dignity, leaving you exposed and vulnerable.

There I was, with a most intimate kind of cancer – one that threatened to take away my breasts and my hair – a cancer that stole my own private body and made it public. Sure enough, friends and family had to comment on my body: what I had done wrong to get cancer, tsk'ing my vanity at my fear of losing a breast or two, commenting on how cancer would cause me to live a "healthier lifestyle" – as if my previous lifestyle was so unhealthy to begin with.

I received an influx of flowers and gifts after my diagnosis, which I am grateful for. I have not forgotten a sentiment or a kind word expressed at that time. The warm thoughts and prayers dried up about a month after my diagnosis.

Then, many people began to abandon me. This weeding out process is natural in the time of crisis, but it was also extremely painful. I lost friends when my first marriage ended and again when Aaron was diagnosed with Down syndrome. The direct rejection of me because I had cancer felt like an arrow through my heart. I couldn't be outraged because I only felt pain.

Add to that, me, the caregiver, had to allow herself to be cared for. My tables had been turned. I'm very grateful that my husband has been my rock. Despite his squeamish nature towards all things medical, he has held my hand through it all.

I've also had flip roles to allow my own children to mother me – and this includes my son with the disability. But to start, telling my three kids that I had cancer was the worst thing I've ever had to do. I hated causing them pain, and this was the rare time that I broke down and cried.

Two weeks after my diagnosis, my daughter, who was 20 at the time and a second-year nursing student, flew out to be with me before my surgery. Her presence was of such comfort to me. She sat down with my husband and me the night before my surgery to review all the materials they had given me to prep. Ella read through all the pamphlets, sharing only the essential information that I needed to know before my partial mastectomy the next day. Mike and I, ages 53 and 48, both professionals who happened to work in health care – Mike in Information Technology, me in Patient Engagement – could not bear to look at the mountains of information that had been given to me up until that point. It was my daughter, a young woman 28 years my junior and deep in her own grief, who stepped up for us.

On the day of my surgery, Mike and I left at 5:30 a.m. for the hospital. Ella helped Aaron get ready for school, dropped him off and then drove into the big city to keep us company. Seeing Ella buoyed my lagging spirits.

She nursed me when I came home from the hospital, calmed me when I freaked out about my sore arm (common after the lymph node removal). In the category of "something a child should never have to do for her mother," she carefully changed my dressings under my arm and on the top of my breast. While her nursing education came in handy for this, it was Ella's kind and gentle nature that helped me begin to heal.

I felt terribly guilty about all of this. I was supposed to be looking after her, as I knew she was in pain and grief too. I think I thought I was strong enough to care for myself, but I simply wasn't. I was weak and vulnerable and in terrible mental shape after my surgery. A chunk had been taken from my breast, and surprisingly, the pain under my arm was awful. I needed Ella and she was there for me, even if I was crabby and down and poorly behaved. She showed me pure and unconditional love.

My eldest son, now 26 and a musician, travelled from his home in the US to visit me in the spring. His presence was greatly anticipated and helped me pass the time waiting for treatment to begin. He did my heart good. We went for ramen and ice cream and he slept in the bottom of his little brother's bunk bed. I tearfully drove him to the airport the next day. He emailed me often.

I am learning to appreciate the people who showed up for me and am working hard to forget those who haven't. I have had exceptional support from my husband and my children. In this way, I am blessed.

My Well-Cared-For Tumour

the challenges of looking into the future when you have cancer

Look at the sky.
We so rarely look at the sky.
– Brother David Steindl-Rast

I n the midst of all this chaos, time marched on. Life didn't slow down because I had cancer. My husband went to work, Aaron went to school, my kids paused but then had to continue with their lives, as they should. I kept trying to return to my book, which I now saw as my job. I'd look at it, befuddled, move a few things around and then shut it down. I simply couldn't think. The book's key messages – health care and kindness – were too close to home.

I was in the middle of experiencing interactions in health care settings that were both kind and unkind. Before, I had over a decade to reflect on interactions in health care that had occurred with Aaron to mold them into stories. The stories that were happening to me as a patient were in real-time. My hospital experiences hit me like assaults and I could acutely feel the sting of care that was dismissive or not compassionate.

I cancelled all my work engagements for the year, not knowing how long I'd be in treatment. I pulled out of an impending talk with a group of pharmacists that was scheduled a month after my surgery. I knew the last thing I could do in my state was to stand up behind a podium and talk about kindness. I needed to erase all the anxiety-provoking people and events in my life in order to survive the days.

I regretted having to leave my job even more fiercely than I had before. If I was going to work three days a week, at least I'd have a distraction (and medical leave and benefits). But the part of my identity that worked in a children's hospital was gone. I was a barely-there wife and mother and only had my dark thoughts to keep me company during the long days. I mostly waited for yet another phone call from a booking clerk or travelled, white-knuckled, to another medical appointment and then counted down the hours until I could fall into bed and go to sleep. Sleep was the only blissful time when I didn't ruminate on cancer or who had abandoned me.

Clinically, I know next to nothing about breast cancer, but I do know a boatload about compassion, respect, kindness and dignity.

I know the little things mean a lot. I know it takes only a minute to ask, "What matters to you?" I know that patients should have information shared with them in a way that they understand. I know the value of a kind touch and a gentle gesture. I know that hospital processes strip away dignity from already vulnerable patients. I know that what is a big deal for patients is often not a big deal to staff. I know that health care inflicts trauma on patients and that staff and physicians should be working hard to minimize that trauma with every single encounter. Most of all, I know that health care professions are intended to be healing professions.

I had the notion that cancer patients were treated well. I think my tumour had been treated very well – and for that I am extremely grateful. I am also thankful to live in Canada, where inpatient hospital costs are publicly funded, and despite the "me-not-working part", our family won't slowly bleed into bankruptcy like my American friends. The one thing I am still not sure about is if I, Sue, as a person, a human being, had been treated as well as my tumour.

How the Little Stuff is the Big Stuff

~ desperately seeking kindness ~

**The essence of who you are is not discovered in your intellect.
It is discovered in your heart.**

– Jean Vanier

T here aren't any staff who have navigator roles where I live, so my dealings were directly with physicians. Navigators can be any professional – nurses, social workers and peer support workers – who are available to patients to help them figure out the cancer world. I wish I'd had access to a nurse or nurse practitioner, but that is not how things are set up in our province. I only had specialists to confer with and they were notoriously guarded by staff who would not let me speak to them directly. I had to wait for my scheduled in-person appointments.

I went to three different cancer physicians in the first three months after being diagnosed with breast cancer.

My first physician was a surgeon who was all business. Yes, I know surgeons aren't famous for their bedside manner and as far as I can tell, she did a fabulous job cutting out the cancer out of my body. People say surgeons can't get emotionally involved with their patients and still be able to cut them open, so I tried my best to understand this. She reviewed my results with me too quickly, but thankfully I saw my family physician a few days later and she translated the pathology and my surgeon's scribbles into a language I could understand.

My second cancer physician was the medical oncologist (shortened to the funny-sounding MedOnc in the cancer world). I mostly saw her resident, not her. This oncologist kept calling me Ms. Robins which was disconcerting and made me feel like she was talking to my mother. She was brisk to the point of being dismissive. I didn't need chemotherapy so she didn't have a lot of time for me and waved my silly questions away. It is true that she had other patients to see who had more serious kinds of cancer, so I tried my best to be understanding of her approach. I took my puny little cancer and slunk away as fast as I could.

My first appointment with the medical oncologist went like this:

My husband drove me to the appointment. I barked at him about something stupid and then apologized, aware I'd been miserable to live with lately. One of my realizations I've had through this whole mess is how deeply this man loves me. For this, I feel terribly lucky. I closed my eyes when we hit traffic gridlock and practiced the breathing I learned at meditation class.

It was a 2.5 hour appointment, but 1.5 hours of that was waiting around sitting on hard chairs in waiting rooms. Everybody was pleasant enough so I don't feel like dissecting this particular patient experience.

It turns out that I have a pathetic kind of breast cancer which replicates at a snail's pace. It could have been brewing in me forever before it escaped my milk ducts and showed up on as a ridge above my heart.

For treatment, I got the best possible news: because my cancer is slow and

the grade is so low, chemotherapy will barely affect my recurrence rate. If
I have chemo, it lowers my recurrence risk by a puny 1%. For me, it is clear
I'm not going to put my family and me through the hell that is chemothera-
py for one percent. So the oncologist prescribes radiation and five years of
estrogen blocking medication for me.

I've been lurching around in shock for months, sometimes so deep in
denial that it felt like a documentary film crew was following me around
recording my fictional life. I took in this news in the same way, numbly,
while my husband kicked into giddy celebration.

I dodged a bullet. There's no reason for this – many good people who are
surrounded by love and prayers and engage in positive thinking and clean
living do not dodge chemo at all. I feel guilty for having such a stupid little
cancer while other women suffer so deeply.

I was a mess after every single one of my appointments, hand-
wringing and second-guessing everything the doctors told me and
ruminating on every word they said for days afterwards. Ask my
sweet husband – I was not fun. Frankly, I was acting like a wounded animal. Eventually, I realized I was struggling to trust what the
surgeon and medical oncologist told me because I did not sense they
cared about me. Well, maybe they did care about me, but they didn't
demonstrate they cared about me.

I dragged my demoralized self to the hospital to meet the third
physician – this time a radiation oncologist. The nurse ushered
anxious me into the clinic room. The first thing the nurse did was
ask me if I wanted a warm blanket. A warm blanket! I love warm
blankets. This appointment was off to an unusual start. My shoulders instantly relaxed and I breathed a bit easier, cozy under my
coveted blanket.

Next, my new doctor knocked on the door and introduced herself
to both me and my husband. She was genuine and lovely. She re-

viewed my pathology results in regular person language, leaning on gardening metaphors and pausing to ask what questions I had. She asked me what kind of writing I did. She patted me on the leg a few times, which gave me great comfort. (There's not enough healing touch in health care. To me, that simple touch gave me a little peek into her caring heart).

She asked me if I wanted to ask my list of questions first, or if I wanted her to explain things and then I could ask any remaining questions afterwards. (I chose the latter). A few times I started to say something and stopped, worried about interrupting her – and she immediately paused and gently said, "Yes, yes, what did you want to say?" She did not appear rushed in any way, even though she had a roomful of patients in the waiting room. She even shared her email address so I could ask any follow-up questions when I got home.

By the end of the appointment, the wounded animal in me had disappeared. The kindness had settled me down. I felt connected to my new doctor and that connection was blossoming into the beginning of trust. This is more than merely being nice – it is about laying the foundation for a relationship.

All the little actions helped to heal my fragile heart – from the warm blanket, the introductions, her gentle approach, her hand on my leg and the way she held space for my questions. All this so-called soft stuff is so much more than just kindness. With her words, gestures and actions, this physician was demonstrating respect and caring too. It was not only what she did, but how she did it.

I might still have had cancer, but I was finally at peace for the first time in a long time. This was because I felt taken care of. These little things may have seemed like nothing to those who work in cancer hospitals, but in my state of heightened vulnerability, they meant just about the world to me.

My Monkey Brain

∽ how cancer affected my mental health ∾

If we knew each other's secrets,
what comforts would we find.
– John Churton Collins

I spent one afternoon at the botanical gardens while I was waiting for radiation treatment to begin. I had my botany book clutched in one hand and my umbrella in the other hand as I wandered around identifying flowering trees in the drippy rain.

In doing this, it struck me that in the weeks since my diagnosis, my world either got very small – about 2.8 cm, the size of my tumour – or very large.

I generally tell stories that have a definitive beginning, middle and end, like writers are supposed to do. Marry that up with a couple of poignant life lessons, and voilà: there's a tidy story I'm happy to slap my name on.

I stopped thinking in tidy stories during that time. I didn't think in complete thoughts, never mind poignant life lessons. My mind jumped around as a jumble of phrases.

- *What did I do to deserve cancer?*
- *Is it going to rain today?*

- *Why is the cancer research building so fancy while the patient treatment centre is so shoddy?*
- *What should we have for dinner tonight?*
- *Why is the breast cancer world so polarized and politicized?*
- *How am I ever going to find a swimsuit now?*
- *Do people know how little of their breast cancer fundraising dollars go into services for actual patients?*
- *I feel guilty for not needing chemo.*
- *When can I go for a walk today?*
- *Why has this been such a shitty year? Everybody told me when I had to leave my job that when one door closed, another door opened. But that door wasn't supposed to be CANCER! It was supposed to be something BETTER NOT WORSE! (I think this a lot).*
- *When is that booking clerk going to call me for my next appointment?*
- *How many days until I see my adult kids again?*
- *Why aren't mental health services offered to newly diagnosed patients?*
- *Why are the Republicans so cruel?*
- *Why can't I motivate myself to work on my book?*
- *Is the new episode of VEEP on?*
- *Why have so many of my so-called friends and family dumped me?*
- *How many steps have I taken today?*
- *Am I over-sharing on my blog?*
- *Why are people with disabilities so devalued by society?*
- *Are the Oilers going to drop out of the hockey playoffs so I can get my husband back again?*
- *How do I accept my new "sick person" identity without getting stuck in being a cancer patient forever?*
- *When is Aaron going to finally get that sleep study?*
- *I need to calm the f*ck down.*
- *Should I delete my Facebook account?*

- *What's with the war metaphors and cancer?*
- *Is radiation going to burn my skin?*
- *Where is the nest of the bald eagles that fly past our window?*
- *Is it too early in the day to have a drink?*
- *Is this Tamoxifen making me sad? Or is this sadness just situational?*

This doesn't even form an inkling of a well-constructed essay. These are clearly signs of a ruminating monkey brain.

Patients are in a similar type of state when they show up at the hospital or doctor's office. It is good for health professionals to pause to understand the extreme stress that patients are often under when they arrive for appointments. It might help explain why we are angry or struggle to ask proper questions. The added stress of going to a medical appointment just compounded my wobbly mental health status.

I was clearly not at my best. I was nearing my worst. My mind was jumping around so much that I couldn't remember anything. I wrote everything down in a little red book that I carried around with me. I could barely form a complete sentence. I was not the strong patient advocate I was supposed to be because it felt like I was walking around with my head stuck in a vise that was slowly being tightened with every passing day.

Author Teva Harrison eloquently termed the phrase "the in-between days" to explain the purgatory that is waiting. I was in the in-between days as I waited for radiation to begin. I was so far from having my shit together, I wondered if my old life was just a carefully curated illusion. I feared this cancer had triggered a mid-life identity crisis.[1]

Patients in the waiting rooms are in the in-between days. I did a lot of waiting between the days. The days I didn't have an appointment, I walked around looking at trees in the rain. I managed to get myself to the clinic or the hospital when I was told, but I was scared when I was there. I was scared that the cancer wasn't all gone. I was scared that there was more cancer. I was scared that after all this was over, the cancer would come back. In a nutshell, I was scared of dying.

When I showed up to appointments, I put on nice clothes and makeup and carefully tucked away my monkey brain. I plastered a polite grin on my face.

Don't let my appearance fool you. For patients like me who seemingly present well, this just means that we fake it well. Inside I was having the biggest existential crisis of my life.

Notes

1. Harrison, Teva, In-Between Days: A Memoir About Living with Cancer, 2016, http://www.tevaharrison.com/in-between-days/

Cease to Love Yourself

〜 on cancer and self-loathing 〜

Believe that you can be salvaged.

– Elizabeth Gilbert

If you struggled loving yourself before you had cancer, imagine how deep in a hole you fall into after you get cancer. All my self-loathing rose to the surface from where I'd deeply hidden it. I could no longer hide behind my tried and true methods that I've honed over the years for covering up the pain. This includes, at various times: not eating, eating too much, obsessive exercising, smoking, drinking, men (note: this was when I was not married), getting caught up in other people's drama, being a codependent partner (in my earlier relationships), and whirling around in anxiety and ruminating thoughts – my current favourite coping-with-pain mechanisms.

Every day I woke up in mental pain. I wasn't sad or angry – I just felt upset all the time. I wished I could cry to at least shed some of the pain.

Now that it was exposed, I couldn't cram the pain back inside.

There was no carpet big enough for me to sweep it back under. I had arrived at my day of reckoning. I had no choice but to do something with it. This is not the silver lining from cancer that I was looking for.

Loving myself has been really difficult to do. I read rah-rah posts on the internet about cancer patients' transformations into strong, courageous people who could do anything. I felt the opposite of this. I felt small. I wanted to disappear. I had no bravado.

It would have been helpful if I had loved myself before I had cancer, but this was now a moot point. I had this strange mix of hating myself, wondering what the whole point of me was, combined with feeling a tinge of self-compassion.

This tinge of compassion was new. This is something I nurtured in therapy. Months of talk therapy helped me.

I've spent my life minimizing my pain and my joy, feeling only those safe emotions straight down the middle – the fear, anxiety, frustration, being upset, feeling outraged – none of the good stuff. I still couldn't cry. My heart was wrapped so tight in my defense, neither sorrow nor joy could get in.

A little tinge of compassion started leaking into my broken heart. Finding a way to love myself would be my salvation. There were months of the dark, confusing and messy. It was the cloud that enveloped me.

I was mad at my body. Arthur Frank's book *The Wounded Storyteller* was a great comfort to me. It helped me understand why I felt betrayed by my body.[1]

Frank talks about the disciplined body-self, which seems like another way to hate yourself. This means controlling your body, engaging in rituals that include adherence to medical care, but also can incorporate strict diet or exercise regimes. No white sugar. No red meat. Go vegan. Train for a marathon, preferably one that supports breast cancer. Imposing discipline on your body is not necessarily loving yourself. This is disassociating from your body to punish yourself.

He notes that cancer treatment is also a regime and many of us express relief when we are finally in treatment. At least something is being done. All we have to do is show up to the hospital and be swept along with the process. It reminded me of a zipline: show up at your appointed time, put on your gear and just step off the platform into the air. There is no talent in ziplining, only the ability to walk off the edge. You must have faith that your harness will support you until you get to the other side.

Frank tells the story of a woman who, after breast cancer, prided herself on returning to work immediately after her mastectomy. She saw cancer as her punishment to bear. Only when she experienced a relapse and decided to end chemotherapy early did she finally break from her regime. It was only then that she made peace with her body and herself.

I stopped taking pleasure in food and drink, so I just ate mindlessly. I felt like the first cancer patient who gained weight. (I know now that weight gain is common for many patients). Then I went on a strict diet for an entire year and lost the weight and more. The dieting was a version of hating my body.

Three years later, I've stopped with the extremes. I walk every day and for the most part, I eat when I'm hungry and stop when I'm full. My body has gotten me through a lot and I'm trying to honour it instead of punishing it. Like many women, this has been a lifelong struggle for me and cancer really didn't help one little bit.

Notes
1. Frank, Arthur, The Wounded Storyteller, 1995, https://www.press.uchicago.edu/ucp/books/book/chicago/W/bo14674212.html

Becoming
a Sick Person

∼ the shift in identity when you become sick ∽

Breathe, darling, this is just a chapter.
It's not your whole story.

– S.C. Lourie

S ome kinds of cancer appear without symptoms. One day we feel perfectly healthy, the next day we are told our cells have become evil and are scheming to kill us. This weird disconnect does not help sudden cancer patients move along the path to acceptance. I never once felt like I had cancer until the treatment began.

Instead, I felt many things: the emotional pain from hurting my immediate family, the abandonment by other family and friends, and the physical pain from surgery and treatment. I never *felt* the cancer. Cancer was like a big joke. For a few weeks, I was certain that I had been over-diagnosed – that my mass was so early stage, so low grade that we really should have left well enough alone, instead of scanning and digging around in my poor innocent breast.

One thing about being told you have a malignant mass in your body – no matter how slowly it is growing – is that this news necessitates some action. It was not suggested that I shouldn't be treated. I was offered a mastectomy, but instead I chose what is termed breast-conserving surgery, also known as a partial mastectomy or a lumpectomy. I was told that chemotherapy would cause more harm than good. In the end, I endured radiation treatment instead. "You are so lucky not to have chemo," many people said to me. Yes, I am the luckiest unlucky person you know.

I never felt sick, except sick in the head. I never felt pain, except pain from people cutting into me and burning me. Cancer treatment remains barbaric and brutal. Patients secretly whisper this vivid description of cancer treatment to each other: slash, poison and burn.

Imagine being in your 40s, minding your own business, considering yourself a relatively healthy person and then suddenly becoming a sick person. Do not underestimate the power of this transition. Being diagnosed with cancer or another serious ailment is a quick-fire path to an identity crisis. This must be an especially befuddling time for patients with no experience in health care. I had the advantage of kind of, sort of, halfway understanding what was happening to me. I'm not sure this partial knowledge is an advantage. It may have been a curse instead.

As a patient, you are put on a conveyor belt of appointments. Your time in between appointments is spent waiting for other appointments. Everything else in your life becomes displaced. The appointments start to define you, for the information shared in those clinic and treatment rooms contributes to your shifting identity. First you are a diagnostic imaging patient, while mammograms, ultrasounds and biopsies ensue. Then if you are unfortunate enough to be diagnosed with cancer, you are a surgical patient. Strangers will discuss with you whether to cut off some or all of your breasts. After that, you are a medical oncology patient, which entails embarking on chemotherapy for some, or taking estrogen blockers for others. You become a radiation oncology patient briefly but only during your time of radiation treatment. Finally, you are back to the world of medical oncology and diagnostics after treatment is done for occasional follow-up appointments. Nobody tells you this whole plan, as the information is doled out one new doctor at a time.

This lurching about the world of specialists is confusing at best. If you've had to step away from your paid work, or enlisted help with caring for your family, even more identity is taken from you. You slowly start to become sick even if you don't feel sick.

March 25, 2017

One month after surgery

The past few months, driving to doctor's appointments is like showing up to my worst imaginable speaking engagement. I haven't adequately prepared, I've left my speaking notes at home, the projector for the slides won't work and the tech guy is nowhere to be found. Worse though, in this case, I'm also standing in front of a hostile audience, like a fool, in a thin blue hospital gown that opens at the back with not a stitch of clothing on underneath.

When patients present to those working in the health system, we are grappling with a lot of this stuff. Throughout my experience, I was hyper-alert during all interactions in hospitals and clinics. This included my touches with receptionists, parking attendants, nurses, physicians and therapists. Nobody missed my gaze. I was both egocentric, thinking that everybody was staring at me, and invisible, knowing that I was yet another generic, middle-aged female cancer patient wandering around the hospital and not worthy of any attention. The cancer hospital is a solemn place. Nobody smiles at you in the hall.

Susan Sontag's famous book *Illness as a Metaphor* compares cancer to tuberculosis, another diagnosis that was used to evoke fear in people's hearts:

> *"...the disease itself (once TB, cancer today) arouses thoroughly old-fashioned kinds of dread. Any disease that is treated as a mystery and acutely enough feared will be felt to be morally, if not literally, contagious. Thus, a surprisingly large number of people with cancer find themselves being shunned by relatives and friends..."* [1]

This is true. A patient presents at the hospital. They are suffering in so many ways: they've been abandoned, they have been shunned, they are in emotional pain, they are in physical pain – often brought about by interventions done at the hospital. They are struggling with their identity, they are worried about their loved ones, they've had to leave their job, they are concerned they won't be done in time to pick up their kid from school, they can't afford the parking fee, they are freaked out that today might bring more bad news and the cloud of death is following them about like they are Pig-Pen from the comic strip Peanuts.

Wherever they are, there's that cloud, cloaking and diffusing everything else. It is nearly impossible to shake, despite desperate attempts at meditation, slow breathing, exercise, mindfulness, positive thinking, gratefulness, medication and trying to calm the fuck down. The cloud of death is ominous, my constant reminder.

Regret comes rushing in: I should have travelled more. Had the discipline to finish that book. Regret for a lost future: I wanted to hold my grandchildren. Be at my youngest child's high school graduation. Regret that I hurt my children when I told them I had this terrible disease.

So you take this person, formerly a regular human being who is now suffering immensely, and morph them into a patient in the hospital. Don Berwick explains this well in a description of a patient, Bert, who is hospitalized:

> "Put him in a johnnie (gown) so his underwear shows. Label his arm. Talk at his bedside as if he weren't there. Put it in Latin. Tell him the visiting rules....If he asks for his laboratory results, tell him you need permission to show it to him, because the numbers might scare him."

He continues on:

> "Yell out 'Bert' in the waiting room, but introduce yourself as 'Dr. Jones', or not at all. Keep him waiting. Keep him guessing. Make him tell you his name, address and phone number five times; make him tell you his symptoms ten times. Take his blood pressure twenty times without ever telling him what it means... Do not ask Bert for his opinion, or his help, or his preferences, or his values, or even his knowledge of himself." [2]

I am poor Bert.

I had to stand obediently at the reception to check in. Line up on the left side of the desk, not the right, or I would (and did) get reprimanded. The receptionist seemed to hold a great amount of authority. It seemed important to get on her good side. I had to cite my cancer hospital number to get any sort of service at all. I was a number.

Once I checked in, I was sent alone down the hall to find the waiting room, which always had a blaring television mounted on the wall, tuned to CNN. In 2017, that meant you had to sit in the waiting room listening to Donald Trump. This was not a peaceful thing to do before a cancer appointment. Sometimes I had to take off some of my clothes before I sat in the waiting room with everybody else. We all sat there like prisoners, in silence in our matching outfits. There was no escape.

None of this seems strange to the people who work at hospitals, for they go to work every day and have stopped noticing these little things. All of this has become normalized, until the inevitable day that the staff themselves become some kind of patient. It is only then that they realize that the view from the other side of the bed is quite stunning.

Notes

1. Sontag, Susan, Illness as Metaphor and AIDS and its Metaphors, 2001.
2. Berwick, Donald M., Escape Fire: Designs for the Future of Health Care, 2003, https://www. amazon.ca/Escape-Fire-Designs-Future-Health/dp/0787972177

There Is Not One
Way to Do Cancer

⌒ searching for meaning in the cancer ⌒

There's no hierarchy of pain.

– Lori Gottlieb

I carried Audre Lorde's book *The Cancer Journals* around in my bag during my cancer treatment. There's so much to admire in her book: her call to women not to be silenced, her refusal to go back to normal and wear a prosthetic to please men or make the nurses in the oncologist's office more comfortable.

> *What are the tyrannies you swallow day by day and attempt to make your own, until you will sicken and die of them, still in silence?*[1]

Then I read Elizabeth Wurtzel's piece on having advanced breast cancer:

> *Everyone else can hate cancer. I don't. Everyone else can be afraid of cancer. I am not. It is part of me. It is my companion. I live with it. It's inside of me. I have an intimacy with cancer that runs deep.*[2]

You may have a strong opinion after reading these quotes. Think about how that strong opinion comes through your own lens about how you think you would handle breast cancer. Remember that how you think you'd deal with cancer is only a guess. You never know how you might actually feel until it arrives.

We all respond to cancer in our own way. Our response depends on our own values, how we have responded to crises in the past and our toolbox of resiliency. Cancer is terribly personal, for cancer is not an external invader. It is our own cells that have turned against us. So that means that a patient's response to cancer is deeply personal too.

Because we are all different, we all do cancer differently. The secret is to never assume how a person might feel. The other secret is that even if you have had cancer yourself, don't assume others experience it in the same way that you did.

When I first got diagnosed, I spoke to many women who had a cancer experience. Each of them told me different things: put your head down and get through it; fuck that shit; be strong; endure so you can get back to your life; here's your chance to be healthier and become vegan. Each had formed their own cancer philosophy which had evolved over time.

I lean towards Audre's outlook instead. She talks about having "survived cancer by scrutinizing its meaning within our lives, and by attempting to integrate this crisis into useful strengths for change."

How could I have not changed? I'm not going back to the way I was before I had cancer. I see that as a waste of all the emotional and physical pain that arrived along with the cancer. But then that's just me. Not everybody feels that way and that's okay too.

My response to having breast cancer was very Sue. I searched for kindness and compassion from my family, friends and health professionals because that's what I've always done. I'm all about the soft stuff, so naturally I looked for it when I got cancer too. I struggle with fitting in and belonging, so I tried many support groups, outlets and cancer-supportive organizations before I found my fit. I grapple with self-worth, so any rejection by family, friends and health professionals devastated me.

I'm a reader, so I read a lot in an attempt to understand how cancer feels. I'm a writer so I wrote about it for many reasons – to bear witness to myself, to offer constructive feedback, to say thank you, to bitch and moan, to collaborate, to heal myself.

I bristled against certain cancer words to describe myself (survivor, warrior) before settling on the neutral breast cancer haver. Now I am a woman who had breast cancer and there's no evidence of it right now but it has a chance of coming back. That's a mouthful but one word doesn't sum me up. Mostly you can just call me Sue.

Since my paid work has been in patient experience, this lens is particularly strong. I was tuned into every aspect of my experience with health care – from how appointments are booked (archaically) to bedside manner (a mix) to the waiting room environments (mostly crappy).

Cancer is an opportunity to lift each other up – even if we don't look or behave exactly alike or have the same diagnosis. Let's give each other permission to be sick – and live life – exactly as we want to, without fear of punishment.

When patient has cancer, it is not about you. It is about them. Be aware of your own values. Suspend judgement. Simply let them live out their own story in the way that feels right to them.

Notes

1. Lorde, Audre, The Cancer Journals, 1980, https://www.auntlute.com/the-cancer-journals
2. Wurtzel, Elizabeth, I have cancer. Don't tell me you're sorry, 2018, https://www.theguardian.com/commentisfree/2018/jan/20/cancer-elizabeth-wurtzel?CMP=share_btn_tw

It Is What It Is

~ a plea to stop blaming the patient ~

**I do think people offer certainties
when they think that you're proof of
something that scares them.**
– Kate Bowler

I breastfed my three kids for six years (not each, sillies, all together) and naively thought that made me immune to breast cancer.
This is an arrogant way to think: to be so pious to assume others
with cancer brought it on themselves and you are somehow above
that because you ran marathons or breastfed your babies or didn't
eat sugar.

Cancer doesn't work that way. That's the problem with risk factors
– they are only factors, not absolutes. And even if this was all my
fault, does that mean I deserve any less treatment or compassion?
Think about that for a moment. If you believe that, I might be able
to sell you a membership to the Republican Party.

When I felt that lump, I didn't become alarmed until the lump
resulted in a mammogram and then an ultrasound and then a biopsy three long months later. And then, sure enough, a diagnosis of
breast cancer followed the next week.

(Note for my friends going through the same process: 80% of biopsies come back benign. If one in nine Canadian women get breast cancer, consider me your "one" out of nine women you know, including yourself. I'm taking that "one" for the team).[1]

Believe me, I've heaped enough blame on myself: I'm curvy and not particularly fit and I do enjoy a regular glass of wine. These are risk factors which, in my darkest hours, I calculated probably wiped out any advantage from all that childbearing and subsequent breastfeeding.

Then I moved to blaming the environment – hormones in my food (but wait, this meant I didn't make healthy food choices – damn) or growing up in oil-loving Alberta, with refinery dust settling on me as I biked to elementary school.

Of course, this is all speculation, also known as the blame part of grief. I went through the same process when my son was born with Down syndrome (my eggs are old and wrinkly! It was the refineries!) to no avail.

As far as a philosophy, a friend who has had a lot of stuff happen in her life, says, equally profoundly, "Shit happens."

Even Science magazine chimes in, saying, "...66% of cancer-promoting mutations arise randomly during cell division in various organs throughout life."[2]

Now I have a son with three copies of his 21st chromosome and I'd never consider him a mistake. I have always felt he has a chromosomal difference, not a disorder, and that he is a part of the natural human fabric just like everybody else.

Me with my cell mutation – well, true, it will kill me if I don't treat it, so that's a problem. But sometimes random shitty things like cancer just happen.

Notes
1. http://www.hopkinsmedicine.org/breast_center/treatments_services/breast_cancer_diagnosis/breast_biopsy.html
2. https://www.sciencemag.org/news/2017/03/debate-reignites-over-contributions-bad-luck-mutations-cancer

Once I Ate a Doughnut

~ reflecting on patient blaming that goes along with cancer ~

Out beyond ideas of wrongdoing and rightdoing,
there is a field. I'll meet you there.

– Rumi

The key message at a two-day workshop for cancer patients that I attended was: *it was your shitty lifestyle that gave you cancer, and if you don't change your shitty lifestyle, your cancer will recur.*

Halfway through day two, I stood up and walked out. If my time here on Earth is limited, I don't need to spend my days being lectured to about this kind of sanctimonious crap.

Instead, I went for a long walk, met my husband for a lunch (I had a salad, just for the record, since I'm feeling defensive about what I eat now), went for another long walk along the beautiful Vancouver seawall and met up with a dear friend for tea. This seemed like a healthier way to spend my time.

I signed up for the workshop a few weeks after my radiation treatment was done. I thought, "I'll show up and be open to learning." I lasted a day and a half before the blaming, finger pointing and judgemental tone of the lectures from the "experts" did me in.

The room was filled with people with cancer who had lived healthy lifestyles. I'd call this the classic West Coast way of life – in this case, there were many fit, nutrition-conscious women who happened to have breast cancer. (And they were pretty pissed off about it, too). There were also three young people whose cancer had recurred.

The presenters did not understand their audience. I'm not sure how blaming people with cancer for getting cancer in the first place is helpful. Patients do not need more fodder to add to our own feelings of guilt. We are also not stupid. We know that being active and eating healthy is important. No kidding.

Even if I smoked, drank, was obese, ate too many doughnuts, warmed up my food in plastic containers in the microwave, does this mean that I deserved to get cancer or that I am less deserving of care or compassion for my cancer?

The idea that getting cancer is a punishment for being bad is particularly prevalent in North American society. Two different people said to me after my diagnosis: Well, maybe you will adopt a healthier lifestyle now. (One of those people had breast cancer themselves – and she tightly controlled her body through diet and exercise. The other was a friend who is vegan and a runner). Of course this sentiment implies that my unhealthy lifestyle is the reason I got breast cancer to begin with.

This "blame the patient" approach is common in health care, too. Every few days, a new article appears in my Twitter feed about exercise preventing breast cancer or relapses in breast cancer. People with lung cancer are blamed, whether they smoked or not. And who cares if they smoked? Does not leading a perfectly controlled life mean you deserve cancer?

This patient-blaming attitude is pervasive everywhere, including in Canada. (Although I'm extremely grateful for our Medicare, which is our quasi-universal health care coverage for hospital and physician office care. This means I don't have to pay for my medical care because I got sick).

The truth: cancer is a combination of genetics, bad luck, rogue cells – and yes, environment and lifestyle are factors too. But there is no one cause of all cancers – cancer is much more insidious than that. Our own cells turn feral on us for all sorts of reasons. If researchers knew what that reason really was, we would already have a cure for cancer. You can't prevent cancer by doing any one thing.

The real reason I think people are blamed for getting cancer is because we are all terrified of becoming vulnerable, needing help and dying. We think that we can do all sorts of things to avoid death. Alas, there is a randomness to living that is out of our control. There was a one in 700 chance I'd have a kid with Down syndrome, but I had him anyhow.

I know I have lived through many women's biggest fear. Once you start with the boob-squishing mammograms, the idea that you might have breast cancer begins floating around in your mind.

I'm not suggesting you don't encourage people to live a healthy life, whatever that means to you. That would just be silly. But...stop the patient blaming when people do get sick. None of us are going to escape this world without acquiring some sort of illness and eventually dying. This is part of life.

My healthy lifestyle changes since getting cancer include: holding those who showed up for me close, more hugging, going to therapy to finally figure out how to love myself, meandering on long walks, marvelling at sunsets and remembering to breathe. I still eat cheese, lie around in my bed watching Netflix and enjoy a tall glass of cider. Everything in moderation, folks. My best advice is to go forth and live your life with joy and not fear.

My message to those cancer workshop organizers is that shaming patients is not going to lead to behaviour change. I have a news flash for all those folks who run marathons, adhere to strict diets and live a virtuous life: this does not make you immune to death. If this control gives you some peace in your heart, I do not judge it. But do not judge me if these aren't tactics that I employ.

Being perfect does not prevent cancer. Treat those who are suffering with respect and compassion. Suspend your pious judgement and meet people where they are at. People who have cancer need your help, not your disdain, to learn how to heal, both inside and out.

Susan Gets Radiated

∽ my first-hand account of radiation therapy ∽

Please, tell me more about
my own goddamn experiences.
–Aaron Reyolds

At 8:15 a.m., I walk into the sad building that is the cancer hospital. So dated and scuffed, the elevator always packed, the piano in the lobby sitting empty. I go upstairs and dutifully wait in line to register. Last time I didn't stand on the left, as the tattered sign instructed me to and I was scolded. This time I know better. "Follow the green line to Treatment Area Seven," I'm told. So that's what I do.

Treatment Area Seven is at the very end of the building. I walk past the other treatment areas and peek into the waiting areas. They are filled with people in various stages of pain.

I'm feeling especially sad for myself because I'm alone.

I get to Treatment Area Seven and sit down. I notice other women there have already changed into gowns. It is only women. I don't know if Treatment Area Seven is just for breast cancer or what. Nobody tells me anything.

I'm not sure if the staff know I'm there. I don't have a gown. I try to ask a woman across from me – "Excuse me," I say, but she is immersed in her phone and doesn't answer. She wears a scarf to cover her bare head and I feel guilty that I don't need chemo. I don't bother her again.

I'm now thinking there's no way they know I'm here because I don't have a gown. So I get up and present myself to Treatment Area Seven's desk. A young man looks up, annoyed. "Just go sit down," he says. "Okay," I say, compliant and small. The TV is blaring a shrill morning news show in the holding area. There's no peace here. I sit and close my eyes.

The same young man calls my name. "Susan," he says. "Call me Sue!" I say cheerfully. "Nobody calls me Susan anymore."

He's still annoyed with me. I must be like 25 years older than him. I am an old woman to him – worse, an old woman with cancer. He has the information he needs to share with me on a wipeable plastic piece of paper. I know after he's done with me, he will just wipe me away.

First he wants to set me straight for coming up to the desk. "Don't come up to the desk," he says. "That interrupts us and we are busy working." I nod like I'm supposed to. "Next time put this pink card in that box so we know you are there." I protest meekly, "I didn't know. It is my first time." He stares at me blankly, like it has never been someone's first time before. "The receptionist just told me to come here," I say finally, quietly.

This seems like a dumb thread of conversation, so I give up, defeated. I hope he's not my radiation therapist because I don't want him to see my scarred and beleaguered breast.

He hands me the pink card with my appointment times for next week scrawled on it. I cannot get over how archaic and paper-based this whole thing is. It is like 1961. What if I lose this coveted card? I'm sure that means I'd be in trouble. I can't help but peek at the times.

Three of out five of them are either early in the morning or late in the day. When they called me last week and asked my preference for time, I said 10 a.m. to 1 p.m. There are only two mid-day times. Immediately I start panicking, thinking about how I'm going to get childcare to get Aaron back and forth to school. Crap.

"Um," I say, hesitant to interrupt his reading of the information from the plastic sheet. "I can't come at these times," I say. I bring on yet more annoyance. "I can talk to the clerk but I can't guarantee it," he says.

I reluctantly pull the disability card. "My son has a disability. Not just anybody can pick him up from school." This is a bit exaggerated but mostly true. I don't know if this helps or just makes me look more pathetic. Patient has cancer AND a kid with a disability. Sad. "We'll see," he shrugs.

I follow him around as he shows me where to get changed. There's some complicated formula for the gown thing – I'm to wear the same one every time so they don't have to wash it as much. I leave it in a numbered bag and hang it back up afterwards. I have to remember my number.

"Okay," I keep saying, nodding. At the end, he says, reading off an invisible script, "If you have any questions, just come and ask us." I am puzzled by this comment. I thought I wasn't supposed to come up and speak to them. Maybe it depends what kind of question I have.

I get changed and look at myself in the mirror. I look terrible. My hair is frizzy. My hair colour is all fading and I look unhinged. My mascara is smudged under my eyes. Why did I bother wearing makeup? I haven't slept much. In fact, I haven't slept much since I found that ominous lump six long months ago.

I sit back down. They call my name again, "Susan". This time I don't bother to correct them. Susan it is. Maybe it can be Susan who has cancer. Sue does not have cancer. I'll go back to Sue later.

The radiation therapists are both women, but they are considerably less warm than the staff who did my CT scan last week. No chit-chat, nothing. "Climb up here," they say. I was going to joke, "This is just like the spa!" but I opt to say nothing. They do not seem like the joking types. They do introduce themselves, but everything they do feels like they are ticking off a box on the list.

I have to hold my breath when I am radiated. I cannot believe how stupid this sounds and how long it took the researchers to figure out that if you have cancer on the left side, holding your breath during radiation helps prevent heart disease. At least I hope it does anyhow.

"At your CT scan, you let some air out while holding your breath," the radiation therapist scolds. Immediately I feel shame. "They told me I did a good job!" I say, lightly. "You let some air out," she repeats Then she produces what looks like a clip to hang clothes. "If you do it again, you have to wear this," she says. I don't want to wear a clip on my nose. I have a recurring nightmare of suffocating underwater because I can't breathe. "I'll do better," I promise.

The lights are blaring above. I wonder why they can't turn them down. I read once there is sometimes music. There is no music here, just the whirring of the machine. I close my eyes. They are yanking the sheet under me to put me in the right position. I pretend I'm sitting on the beach. I imagine watching the waves flow in and out. I keep breathing. I think, "Someone should teach patients relaxation techniques before they start treatment." I have to work more on relaxing. Right now, I'm the least relaxed person on Earth.

They exit the room and I'm alone with the machine. I already hate the machine. This is the coldest and least human kind of health care. I crack open a tiny bit and start crying. My hands are above my head, in some sort of weird S&M position and I can't wipe away my tears. I can't cry and hold my breath at the same time, so I'm a bit panicked. I have to calm the fuck down.

They talk to me through an intercom. Apparently there's a video camera on me so they probably saw me crying but they don't care. I wonder if other women cry. The faceless voice instructs me over the speakers. I have to take deep breaths in and hold them for a long time. I am obedient, scared of getting the nose clip and try to comply. My poor left breast is exposed, both to the air and to the burning radiation rays. Slash, poison, burn. That's cancer treatment in a nutshell.

I feel nothing now, but later, my skin will be burned. It is cumulative so I'll be scorched after a few more sessions.

It is done. I don't know how long it took. Maybe 10 minutes? I get off the table and stand awkwardly in the room. "You can go," they say, pointing to the exit. "Thank you," I say. I thank everybody for doing their job. I know this game. If I'm not overly grateful, I'll be labeled as difficult, which won't help if I need a favour one day.

I need to ask about my appointment times, but there's that guy sitting at the desk again. I march back up there, taking my chances. I need my pink card back.

He's busy using liquid paper of some sort to change the times on my card. Now only one is not mid-day instead of three. "Thank you so much," I say, again. I see the door across the hall says, "Radiation booking clerk" so I know this hasn't been much effort for him.

I get changed and get the hell out of there, following the green line all the way back to the elevator. I can't figure out where the stairs are, so I stand silently in the full elevator for only one stop, looking at the floor.

I sit alone in the cafeteria with a tea, waiting for my Mike to arrive. He is rushing to get here after dropping Aaron off at school this morning. One burn down, 19 more to go.

(Note: I wrote this essay after my first day of radiation. I had 19 more sessions of radiation treatment, but this first one was definitely the worst and the one I remember the best).

The Tale of Two Appointments

∽ contrasting two medical appointments – one kind, one unkind ⌒

The world's deepest wound is not being understood.

– Pico Iyer

I had two separate diagnostic imaging appointments. One was for an ultrasound at the cancer hospital and the other was for a follow-up mammogram at a diagnostic imaging centre. Both appointments involved my poor breasts, but otherwise the two experiences could not have been more different.

I sat in my therapist's office afterwards and deconstructed each appointment. I'm figuring out why I am so desperate for kindness in health care settings. A chunk of that is my own stuff – I seek comfort when I'm feeling vulnerable. But no matter my own personal reasons, I hope we can all agree that being mean to people in hospitals and clinics is not an acceptable option.

I present these two experiences to demonstrate how easy it is to be kind, how it does not take more time and how kindness is up to individuals and lack of kindness cannot be blamed on the "system". Never forget the system is made up of people. Even in a health care culture that does not promote kindness for its own staff, there is opportunity for exceptional folks to go against culture to demonstrate caring for those they've committed to serving.

Example 1: The Ultrasound

I waited among the bank of chairs in the hall, the first appointment of the day. A gentleman pushing a laundry cart called down the hall to me, "Hello there!" This perked me up and made me smile – scared, anxious me, sitting alone in the cancer hospital for my first post-cancer treatment scan. Hello there mattered.

A man came out of the ultrasound room. A man to do my breast ultrasound! But he had a warm smile and called me by name. "Come and get changed," he said, "and I'll meet you in the room. Put the gown on with the back open," he added before he disappeared. I was greeted warmly and clearly told what to do. I appreciated the option of the gown. (This will make sense as you read my other experience). I changed and went into the room. The lights were darkened and there was soft classical music playing. The environment was comforting.

The whole ultrasound took about half an hour. This nice man talked to me the whole time. He asked about my cancer treatment in a conversational kind of way. He told me what he was doing as he was doing it and also shared with me what he was doing next. Providing information about what was happening and what to expect next was a great comfort.

He said, "This might hurt. Tell me if you feel pain." He also said, "I'm almost done" as he was wrapping up. He told me when he left the room and why. He wasn't afraid to acknowledge my pain.

I was still wound tight as a top, clearly worried that all my cancer wasn't gone. He said to me, "Don't be worried." I knew full well he wasn't allowed to tell me anything about my scan. The results of the ultrasound would be faxed to my oncologist in a week (alas, it is the

SUE ROBINS

holidays, so I wouldn't find out the results until the new year). But his "don't be worried" validated my concern and was actually sweet. He lessened my anxiety with his words.

I walked out feeling okay. It wasn't *what* this man did – it was *how* he did it. And none of it took more time. And, surprisingly to me, it did not matter one bit that he was a male technologist because of his compassionate approach.

And then, one hour later, in sharp contrast, I experienced the cold, the officious, the not-so-kind experience.

Example 2: The Mammogram

I had a mammogram earlier that month, but had been called back for another appointment. I asked the booking clerk when she phoned, "Why do I have to come back?" She said she didn't know. So I spent sleepless nights thinking they found more cancer. Not telling me why I had to come in again seemed cruel.

My husband, having dropped Aaron off at school, met me at this appointment. We sat in one crowded waiting room until I was called into another waiting room. On the door it said: *Women only.* No men were allowed. My husband sat on a bench outside the elevator for the next hour. Not permitting my partner to accompany me is not patient or family-friendly.

I sat in the second waiting room for a long time. I was hoping I wouldn't get the same technologist as before, as she was unfriendly. (Irony alert: having a woman technologist does not guarantee a good experience). It turns out I got another woman, who was equally as unfriendly. I knew then unfriendly was the culture of this diagnostic imaging centre, and only the most exceptional clinicians would rise above it.

Then there was the sign that said:

Dear Patients,

We no longer routinely change patients into gowns unless they are having additional exams.

*We hope this improves our **efficiency** and reduces our environmental impact.*

The option for a gown is available if preferred.

I knew to expect it because I had been there before, so I was wise to them. I brought a cardigan to wear in the mammogram room. At my last appointment, I had to strip from the waist up in front of the technologist and stood there, unnecessarily exposed, cold and topless. This time I brought my own cover-up.

There's so much to say about this sign. First, the idea of being efficient by not encouraging gowns is baloney. I sat in the waiting room for 40 minutes. Forty minutes is plenty of time to change into a gown, isn't it? And for environmental impact? Yes, I guess doing laundry is bad for the environment.

All my years of hating hospital gowns and I never would have guessed their solution to sterile gowns would be to take away the gown.

Yes, I could have taken a gown but this was clearly not encouraged. There were other signs too, saying no cell phones. There was a stereo on the floor, tuned into a Christmas music radio station that played loud commercials and cut in and out as people walked past. The room was packed. All of us women were lined up, our fear palpable. Signage and physical space set the tone for the whole patient experience.

Once I was called in, I had to strip from the waist up. I put my cardigan back on and pulled it tightly around me. The woman did not introduce herself. She did not tell me what she was going to do. I said casually, "It is too bad we don't have gowns." "Gowns just get in the way," she responded. Oh. Dignity starts with giving options to minimize patient nudity. (Do I really have to say this?).

I don't want to discourage women from getting mammograms,

but this mammogram hurt a lot. She did tell me they wanted a closer picture of one part of my breast – which happened to be in an awkward position – close to under my arm. I was jammed into the mammogram machine. I whimpered as she tightened the machine around my breast – this one, my cancer side, still swollen with lymphedema from my lymph node removal. She did not acknowledge my pain and clamped down on it some more. Not acknowledging pain does not help with suffering – in fact, it increases it.

She must have taken ten more images. Each time it hurt more. I tried to breathe but I was told to hold my breath. I was starting to feel dizzy and clammy. I had no idea when she would be done. Being left in the dark about what's going on is anxiety-provoking in an already anxiety-provoking situation.

Suddenly, it was mercifully over. I stood in the corner, my back turned and got dressed. I was told to sit in the waiting room again, but I didn't know why. Another woman came about 20 minutes later and told me I could go. I wasn't informed what was to happen next or when my test results would be shared with me. I got out of there as fast as I possibly could.

I met my husband in the hall and he enveloped me in a hug. "What took so long? Did they find something?" he asked, clearly alarmed. I shook my head and said, "just please take me home."

I know how to speak up. I also know how to submit a complaint but I have to say – a lot of good that's done me in the past. Sometimes all we can do is put our head down and endure horrible situations. I don't always feel like being an advocate. I am not always strong. That's ok too.

But I hope I have demonstrated with these stories how a compassionate health professional can make a difference. That the little things matter. That what is not a big deal for health professionals (like topless patients) might be a big deal for us.

Those who work in health care can make a hard situation better by demonstrating compassion. For my whole mammogram experience, all I can say is, I know you can do better.

Anne Lamott says these are the two best prayers she knows: *Help me help me help me. And thank you thank you thank you.* For the ultrasound technologist, I say, thank you. Thank you for making things a little bit easier for a scared, traumatized woman with breast cancer. What you did mattered. In fact, all those so-called little things you did – that took no extra time at all – mattered to me a lot. For you, I am tremendously grateful.

Cancer Care Criticisms

~ what it feels like to be a number in the health care system ~

To do things right, first you need love, then technique.

– Antoni Gaudi

I naively thought there was some sort of gold standard for care when I got cancer. In the back of my head, I thought, "I've hit the health care jackpot! Finally, I will experience the kindness and compassion that I've been seeking all my life." I was wrong.

My care was uncoordinated and disjointed. I jumped from my family physician to diagnostic imaging to more diagnostic imaging to a hematologist to a women's breast clinic to my family doctor to a surgeon to nuclear imaging to day surgery to a medical oncologist to a radiation oncologist to radiation treatment and back to a medical oncologist. Throw in time with a therapist at the cancer hospital, a therapist in private practice and then a psychiatrist, and back to the medical oncologist. Start the cycle up again when I go for a mammogram and ultrasound for my check-ups.

In all, my appointments took me to 13 different locations to see over 30 clinicians. This does not include the countless receptionists, technicians, parking staff, cafeteria workers and booking clerks that I encountered along the way.

I didn't even have chemotherapy. Except for my bleeding disorder, which demanded stops at a hematologist, I had a straightforward course of action for my breast cancer. The whole experience was a mess.

Traumatized me drove myself to many of these appointments in the big city. I Google mapped where I had to go and scoped out parking beforehand. I'd search office lobbies and hospital hallways for the appointed room. I'd present myself to the receptionist, anxious and visibly nervous. Did I feel safe? No I did not, not even for a second.

I've been chastised by receptionists for standing in the wrong line, for being three minutes late, or for not having my cancer hospital identification ready. I was standing there eagerly in front of the desk, hoping for some kindness. I felt like a little puppy who has been kicked. The person behind the desk rarely made eye contact with me. Maybe it is too hard to look at someone with cancer? Then perhaps you are in the wrong job. The baristas at the coffee shop are much friendlier to me than you are.

Often the interactions would be brief – name? ID? Date of birth? Sit down. I'd shuffle to the waiting area and sit, head down, with the rest of the downtrodden people with cancer. The chairs were hard. The walls were empty or decorated with hospital posters tacked onto the wall. The magazines were old. The space was eerily quiet, save for an occasional cough. That meant we could hear everything that was said at the reception desk. We'd all jump whenever the nurse appeared to call someone's name. A waiting room in a cancer clinic is the saddest place in the world.

Could the waiting room experience be improved? Why yes it could, only in about a thousand ways. If you sense sarcasm in my tone, you are correct. The waiting room experience is exceedingly simple to fix. But few people seem to care enough to do it.

You can fix it even if you are in an old building and don't have much funding. Where do all those funds go from people who donate to cancer care anyhow? I have never figured that out. Not into patient comforts.

At my medical oncologist's, the first thing that happened was I had to step on the scale. This is a horrible way to start an appointment. "Don't tell me how much I weigh," I'd say, my eyes tightly closed as I stood on the scale. I know damn well if I've lost or gained weight by the way my clothes fit. Why not just ask me? Why do you have to weigh me? I have a feeling it is because that's just the way things are done.

Next, be ushered to the exam room, if you are lucky. Often I'm just told to go to "room 12 and put on the gown." Here's how it typically goes: I find my way there and take off my shirt and bra, and put on the thin hospital gown. I sit in the bare room alone until I hear a knock on the door and in comes my fully-dressed oncologist. (Sometimes it is a family doctor. Other times a resident. I'm never sure who is going to come in because nobody tells me). If it is a new person, I try my best to make a good impression. I'm friendly and I ask about how they are doing. I have my list of questions in my notebook. I obediently allow my breasts to be examined and am often left sitting there nude from the waist up while they talk to me. Despite the fact that it feels like everybody in the hospital has seen my scarred boob by now, it is still embarrassing. My dignity is not intact.

I haven't even gotten to the actual interaction with the physician yet. This physical space and process stuff matters. I don't need a shiny new building with waterfalls and natural light.

I am not looking for hotel service. I am looking for small gestures that comfort patients who are suffering.

Here's what I need: Customer service training for reception staff. Look up. Make eye contact. Don't be distracted. Give the person your full attention, even for 30 seconds. Say hello. Be warm. Chitchat. Use my name. Don't shout personal information all over the waiting room. Smile. Please smile. I'm desperate for a smile to make it okay.

When the nurse calls me in, could she chat with me in the hall and use my name? Could she put her hand on my arm and say it is nice to see me? Could she take me right into the treatment room and not weigh me? Could I be given a gown to preserve my dignity? Could the gowns be soft and patterned like nice pajama tops?

Am I asking too much?

Off My Rocker

∽ my plea to see the both me and my tumour ⌒

I wonder how many people I've looked at all my life and never seen.

– *John Steinbeck*

My tumour was efficiently cut out, disposed of and any remaining cells were bombarded by radiation. I only wish that the rest of me was treated as well as my tumour was.

I know that health professionals know the research about the connection between mind and body. That stress causes illness. That stress does not help with healing. Ideally, yes, I should be the one figuring out how to relax and care for my own mental health, but as a cancer patient, I might need some help doing this. Trying to dig around to find mental and emotional support while I am waiting for and attending cancer treatment is in itself stressful. Do you see the irony there? More suffering is caused by not acknowledging my mental health.

The cancer hospital cares about medical care for my tumour. During an early oncologist appointment, a nurse asks me some routine mental health questions. Do I feel like harming myself? Can I sleep at night? I know how to answer these questions so I would get the help that I needed. Soon I have a referral to counselling services in my hot little hands.

It takes three weeks to get an appointment with a therapist at the hospital. I am only allowed four appointments in total in the public system. If I want more help, I have to switch over to the private mental health system. As a self-employed person, I have to pay for a private therapist out of my own pocket. Luckily, I can afford it. And what of those who cannot? My journal entry a week after my breast cancer surgery begins, "I'm circling the drain here."

Dutifully, I attend my four allotted sessions with the therapist. She validates that what I'm feeling is within the realm of normal. Cancer has revealed all the unresolved pain in my life. Four therapy appointments don't even touch this.

I go to all the publicly-funded stuff I can find. I attend a support group with the national cancer society. I show up to the evening meeting one dark night about three weeks after my surgery. Because the partial mastectomy also took out three lymph nodes, under-neath my arm is killing me but I drag myself into the middle of Vancouver to a boardroom across from the cancer hospital. Note to all organizers: patients do not like attending sessions at or near the cancer centre. Many of us have post-traumatic stress disorder from our treatment and would rather never return, especially for a "sup-port group" session. Just think about how that would feel.

I'm yearning to meet other women who have been through what I'm going through. I show up nervously. The other women seem to know each other, but they are pleasant, smiling at me. Some-one gives me a coupon for the Gap, which is a nice thing to do. The woman who facilitates the two-hour session begins the meeting by telling her own breast cancer story. For half an hour. She had breast cancer seven years ago.

This sets a strange tone. The group goes around the table, each taking a turn to tell their own stories. I'm one of only two new people there and because of the direction of the roundtable, the other new person and I go dead last. There is only ten minutes left for the two of us, so we have to rush.

We have a lot of time to listen to the other women's stories. It turns out all of them have had mastectomies or double mastectomies and they think anybody who hasn't had a mastectomy is a damn fool. "Just cut them off!" one of the women says, referring to her breasts. I am sitting there with my little partial mastectomy, shrinking lower and lower in my chair. I wonder if I can slip out, but the group is small and I feel too Canadian and polite. One of the other facilitators was an oncology nurse, so she starts grilling me about my surgery. She's asking me for details I don't want to share. I start mumbling and pass onto the next woman, who seems horrified too. Thankfully the "support" group has run out of time.

The other newbie and me literally run out of the building and stand in the rain, in the dark, on the street. "Well, nice to meet you," I say. Later, I sit in my car for a long time before I start driving. I am trying to unpack what my panic was about. Part of it was feeling pre-judged for not getting a mastectomy. I hate feeling judged. I can attribute the rest of my feelings to a deep shame. Why did I feel as if I had to defend my stupid little partial mastectomy? Isn't every patient different? Don't we all try to make the best decisions for ourselves at the time?

There were so many ways this support group went wrong. Maybe it was too soon after my surgery to go out in public. Maybe they could have booked a neutral location, far away from the cancer hospital. Maybe the facilitators could have been trained in listening and holding space for the participants, instead of being immersed in their own stories. Maybe the roundtable could have allowed the newbies to tell their stories near the beginning, instead of being rushed at the end. Maybe the "newly diagnosed"' should be separated from the "long-ago diagnosed". Maybe the facilitators could have set some ground rules about being open-minded, and gently explained that everybody makes their own decisions about surgery and treatment for their own reasons.

Maybe I just have to travel on this stupid breast cancer journey all on my own. Maybe I will never call this a "journey" again. It isn't a journey. It is just shit. The two women I knew who I spoke to about their own breast cancer treatment many years ago basically told me to roll up my sleeves and just get it done. How breast cancer feels seemed to have faded away from their memory. Breast cancer was relegated to a simple, chronological story.

I failed miserably at finding my own peer support. I felt so alone but I kept looking.

A colleague of my husband's had just finished up her own cancer treatment. She heard of my predicament. Her initial reaction to my husband's email with my news was perfect. "FUCK," she wrote back to him. She emailed me to set up a coffee. I was a week post-surgery. I showed up to the Starbucks at the mall, weary and sore.

She was a straight-shooter. She told me, "Things are shitty but then some things are good. Try to say, this is shitty but then this is good." This was sound advice. She had chemotherapy and was traumatized about losing her hair. I did not yet know my treatment plan and didn't know that I wouldn't be getting chemotherapy. I listened to her. She was matter-of-fact, but kind.

A few days later, she handed my husband an envelope to give to me. Inside was a note with a little necklace of clasped hands.

These helped me when I was going through all that shit.

This was all the peer support that I had, but maybe this was all the peer support that I really needed.

A Good Therapist

~ why psychosocial oncology is so terribly important ~

Humpty Dumpty sat on a wall,
Humpty Dumpty had a great fall;
All the king's horses and all the king's men
Couldn't put Humpty together again.
– Mother Goose

I t took me time to find the right therapist. After finishing my allotted counselling sessions at the cancer hospital, I started digging around for another therapist who understood cancer.

I have been to therapy before. After my first marriage broke up, I fell into what was termed situational depression which was basically a feeling of being overwhelmed because I was suddenly a single mother of two young children. I had no job and was soon going to have no car or place to live once I finished paying for my divorce. This threw me in a state of paralyzed fear every minute of every day. I only found solace in yoga, walking and my therapist's office.

I had no money, but luckily I found a subsidized program at the local university where a therapy student practiced on me. Sometimes the student's instructor eerily watched us through a two-way mirror. It was a relief to talk to someone who did not give me incessant advice, like my well-meaning friends did.

I went into therapy again when I got remarried. My brand new husband and I went to couple's therapy. I had finally met someone who offered me unconditional love, but Mike and I were not without our troubles. We were madly in love and didn't have relationship troubles with each other, but we did have troubles swirling wildly around our relationship, like ex-spouses and the blending of our families.

When the cancer came years later, I knew I needed help. I was broken in a million pieces and did not know how to put myself back together. It was a real Humpty Dumpty situation that warranted professional help.

After radiation was done, I was looking down the barrel of empty days, five days a week. I filled my time sitting in darkened cinemas watching comedy movies, a smile occasionally escaping from my face.

Mostly, my head was filled with thoughts of my own worthlessness. I thought over and over again, "What's the point of me?"

September 8, 2017

Mike is going out for drinks after work and I've been leaning towards a deep depression every evening, so I fear myself today. Last night I was so down, not anxious, but in a very dark place about myself and that scared me.

I found a therapist at a place that promised a healing space. On their website, there were words like spirit, gentle, deeply rooted, human, soothed. This approach fit me like a glove. My therapist's name is Susie and I'm Sue. I still see her once a month.

The reason I needed therapy during and after cancer treatment was because I had to share the terrible things that had happened to me. I needed help moulding these terrible things into stories so I could start to heal.

There was so much: how cancer had affected me. Fearing death. The betrayal of my body. The medical post-traumatic stress that came from painful diagnostics and treatment. The reason behind why I was always looking for kindness. How cancer disrupted all my relationships. My guilt at causing my children pain.

At first, after I was diagnosed, my days were filled up with appointments at the cancer hospital and the accompanying existential dread. But once cancer treatment ended, all my issues that I had tried to avoid my whole life suddenly surfaced. It was as if cancer had dumped all my unresolved crap onto my kitchen table. My own issues just sat there looking at me, relentless and unblinking.

Many of my troubles came from not liking myself that much. I minimized any pain I felt, dismissed difficult feelings and was not able to feel joy. I had a deep fear of rejection. I felt as if I needed to be a good girl in order to be loved. All these gross feelings were living right in the middle of my belly as I ruminated about all the people who had abandoned me when I got cancer. The abandonment piece was particularly hard.

I needed to look at each of my broken pieces before I could begin to heal. Thankfully that's what therapists are for. My therapist's office was the only place in health care that I could confess I wasn't fine. At the oncologist office, I quickly found that I had to stick to the facts about my physical body. Nobody wanted to hear about my feelings there. They didn't want my story. They only wanted my facts and data.

In Canada, while oncology appointments are covered by Medicare, most mental health services are not publicly funded. We don't have extra health insurance, so I had to pay out-of-pocket to see my therapist. This is expensive and means that accessing a good therapist is only for people who have money. This is not the way it should be.

Since when is your brain not part of health care? My head is still (loosely) screwed onto my body. It is ludicrous that mental health is not seen as an essential medical service and that it is therefore not funded by our government. Mental health services shouldn't only be for the elite. There's much inequity in that. I could afford to go to the therapist only because I was a fortunate privileged person.

Susie was the one person who said to me, "This is hard, this sucks, but it is totally normal to feel this way after cancer treatment ends." Having a person I can openly talk to is one of things that has saved me. Mental health services should not be a luxury for any cancer patient.

Not Dead Yet

∽ side effects and the whole quality of life thing ⌒

I'm sorry your boobies tried to kill you.

– Kim Peschier

There is more to cancer than just not dying.

I asked my radiation oncologist, "How do you know that the radiation treatment worked?"

"When you are alive in twenty years," he bluntly said. And there it was. Above all else, oncology does not want me to become a statistic in their morbidity and mortality tables.

I don't want to die either. But I want to be in decent enough shape that I can live well, for however long that may be. This means taking into account the trauma that is inflicted to our bodies during treatment and the healing that happens after cancer treatment ends.

Cancer is like meeting a stranger with a knife in a dark alley. The stranger says, "I'm gonna mess you up bad," and proceeds to do just that – slashing, cutting, poisoning, burning you through the dark night and into the break of day.

Cancer causes a wave of events in health care environments – diagnostics, diagnosis, treatment. Things happen to you. You ride that wave willingly, eager to rid yourself of the scourge. Once it is all over, all you are left with is you. It was your cells that turned on you. Your own body tried to kill you. It messes with more than your body, it flips your mind upside down. What does it mean if your body tries to kill you?

If we move beyond cancer treatment to cancer care, this means considering a patient's mental, emotional and spiritual health, and physical health. This means not dismissing side effects of treatment or medications as minor or rare – when in fact they can be life-altering. As with the rest of health care, what isn't a big deal for clinicians is often a big deal for patients.

Since my cancer was feeding off estrogen, I was automatically placed on an estrogen-blocking drug called Tamoxifen. The ingestion of this daily pill immediately gave me strong menopause-like symptoms: energy-draining hot flashes and unwanted abdominal weight gain. More ominous symptoms began to appear: my joints were so sore that I could barely get out of bed in the mornings. I was tired. My toenails started to fall off, which was minor, but weird and disturbing. I was turning into a zombie.

If you Google Tamoxifen, you will find blogs and patient discussion boards filled with the horrors of the pill. Other women don't experience side effects at all, save for the occasional hot flash.

I'm not offering medical advice here, but I do wish the medical folks were more forthcoming about the bad side effects. Both an oncologist and a pharmacist briefly spoke to me about taking Tamoxifen. It was just assumed that I would take it. They shrugged off the side effects, as I think they wanted me to be compliant, to ingest the pill, to not scare me off.

A few weeks into Tamoxifen, a dark cloud started to follow me around. This is when my *"What is the purpose of me?"* thoughts began to pop up. This sense of worthlessness sunk in deep. The only things that brought me back from the edge were my therapy appointments and the idea of not wanting to cause my family more pain.

I mentioned these mental health side-effects at my next oncologist appointment. The physician listened to me, her eyes growing big. She excused herself and came back after consulting with a colleague.

"I think you should go off Tamoxifen for a month and see how you are feeling," she offered. She also gave me a referral to a psychiatrist.

It seems that I had gotten their attention. Falling off toenails? Not so much. Despondent thoughts? Yes. I had to be standing right on the edge of a cliff to elicit some sort of response.

Two weeks after stopping Tamoxifen, its effects began to leave my body. Agitating hot flashes disappeared. My pants felt a bit looser. Stopping Tamoxifen just to halt weight gain seems like a vain reason to expose yourself to more cancer risk. But maybe if it helps you feel less crappy about yourself, that's okay. Taking the pill or not taking the pill are intensely personal decisions.

One morning, two weeks after I stopped the medication, I woke up and the pit in my stomach was gone. I had tried so many things to get rid of it: meditation. Walks. Therapy. Was this just a coincidence, a sign of my natural healing? I can never say for sure. The casually dismissed side effects of this nasty drug were real to me. Tamoxifen had caused me more suffering.

Now I was in a pickle. Did I want the cancer to come back? I was supposed to take Tamoxifen for five years to prevent recurrence. But what if I spent those five years in misery? How was that for a quality of life, me dragging my husband and children down into my well of pain? This seemed not okay.

My oncologist was unhappy when I told her that I wasn't going to swallow the little pill again. I decided to take my chances. I needed to focus on healing so I could live my best life. Cancer showed me that I don't have as much time on this earth as I thought I did.

Seeing the Caregiver's Suffering

∿ patients suffer but families do too ∾

We tell ourselves stories in order to live.

– Joan Didion

I f I didn't feel heard as a cancer patient, imagine my dear husband. He was the one who accompanied me to oncology appointments. He was my stabilizing force during my entire cancer experience.

Mike sat in the corner of the clinic room for my appointments, his eyes respectfully averted while I inevitably sat on the examination table topless, my breasts being prodded and poked. I do not ever remember anybody asking him how he was doing. Was his suffering seen? Mine was not; his was seen even less. He was invisible beyond a perfunctory introduction and handshake with the doctor.

Families are interwoven like a baby mobile. If you move one part of that mobile, all the other parts will move around in different ways too. After treatment was all done, Mike confessed to me that my suffering caused him emotional pain. This is because we love each other. I regret that I was so caught up in how I was feeling that I had forgotten about him.

He has his own story as the husband of a woman with cancer. That is his story to tell, not mine.

What I do know is that Mike, who was my greatest cheerleader, love and friend, had transformed into my caregiver. He'd slip away from work and appear in waiting rooms, hunched over in his own pain from my cancer. His face never failed to brighten when he saw me emerge from the change room in my hospital gown. Afterwards he took me for long lunches of ramen or sushi, encouraging me to eat my favourite foods. He would fetch Aaron from school when I could not. He stayed with me and stroked my hair when I was deep in depression. Still, he sat in the corner at every single one of my appointments, quiet and unseen.

How I wish he had been acknowledged in those appointments. A simple, "What questions do you have, Mike?" or "How are you handling things, Mike?" would have honoured the role he has in my life.

Mike kept on loving me when I was struggling with the new emotions that came with cancer: worthlessness, despondency and fear. He had my back at all times. He was my rock. His role in my life was worth at least acknowledging by some simple chitchat in the clinic room.

We have an emptying nest in our home. My two eldest adult children have their own lives far away. I kept in close touch with them, by texting, email and FaceTime. I do not wish to revisit the time I had to call them both to tell them that I had cancer. No mother wants to inflict pain on their children, but that's exactly what my cancer did.

Aaron is our last child at home. He was 13 when I was diagnosed. Nobody truly understands cancer, not those with PhDs or teenagers with an intellectual disability. I firmly told him that he could not catch cancer from me and that it was not contagious. Nonetheless, months later, when he was in the doctor's office for strep throat, he looked at me wide-eyed and whispered, "Do I have cancer?" That broke my heart.

In my 20 days of radiation treatment, I dropped Aaron off at school and dutifully drove across the city to the cancer hospital for treatment. I'd then pick him up from school in an increasingly exhausted state. I tried to explain what "radiation" was (a big x-ray that killed the bad cells) but thought it would be good for Aaron to actually see where I was going every day.

I told the radiation therapy staff that I was bringing my son – who had Down syndrome – with me to my next visit. Mike took the day off work and all three of us arrived at my appointment. The radiation therapist was wonderful – she showed Aaron the machine that delivered radiation and explained how it worked to zap the cancer cells.

After my treatment, I walked down the hospital corridor with Aaron. "What did you think?" I asked.

"It looked like a horror movie," he said, hushed, his head down, clearly disturbed. Damn. I'm not sure bringing him to the cancer hospital was a good idea after all. The real-life image of that huge radiation machine was worse than anything he could have dreamed up in his imagination.

Cancer had invaded all of our lives. Acknowledging both the patient and their loved ones is a big part of patient and family centred care. If a family member shows up at the hospital, this is an opportunity for health professionals to provide a listening ear, offer resources and recognize how difficult cancer can be on the whole family. Cancer really is a family affair.

What Heals Us

it is not what you do, but how you do it
– lessons from a radiation oncologist

Do not look for healing at the feet
of those who broke you.
– Rupi Kaur

I t is a commonly held notion that patients will only give feedback when care is either very bad or very good. Those who have ordinary experiences do not usually take the time to write a letter or fill out a comment card. I'd like to commit to speaking up when things go well and when they go poorly. Here's my story of a perfectly ordinary appointment.

I had time booked with a radiation oncologist at the cancer hospital. I think appointments with oncologists strike fear into most people. It must be a strange job to be an oncologist and have people show up in your office terrified to see you.

This was my first time back at the cancer centre since my last day of treatment. On the drive there, I was an anxious mess. I drove as fast as I could in bumper-to-bumper Vancouver traffic and loudly played a Tragically Hip live album on the car stereo to give me some moxie.

Courage, my word
It didn't come, it doesn't matter
Courage, it couldn't come at a worse time

My regular radiation oncologist was on holidays, so I was booked in to see someone new. I woke up in the morning awash with anxiety thinking about this new doctor. What if he wasn't kind? And yet another new person looking at my poor boob and this time a man to boot? Great. I might as well be marching through the cancer centre with no shirt on with the amount of dignity I had left. I had to go to the appointment by myself, as my husband had to remain at home to look after our son. Being alone never helps my monkey brain either.

I eyed my bottle of Ativan before I left. Isn't it ironic that the main reason I pop anti-anxiety pills is when I have an appointment at the hospital? I decided instead of taking a pill to park a few blocks away from the cancer centre and walk to see if the trek would help settle me down. (It did).

I hiked through the leafy residential neighbourhoods, grabbed an iced coffee and snuck in the back through the parkade elevator. The sight of all the people with cancer waiting in the lobby always makes me sad. In fact, the whole building makes me sad. It isn't my favourite place to go.

I dutifully checked in with the receptionist, who was pleasant enough, and sat down for about three minutes before my name was called. I have to say that the radiation folks are all very efficient – there's very little waiting in that department. The nurse (I think?) who fetched me asked how I was doing. She didn't share her name or her role and I didn't have the energy to ask. We chatted a bit about burned boobs and fatigue and she left me alone in the room to change into a gown. The radiation oncologist knocked and came in a few minutes later.

He was a young physician with a gentle manner. He introduced himself and shook my hand. He sat down in the chair while I was perched on the treatment table. I knew this was my last radiation oncology appointment and so I had my notebook with my list of questions for him.

In total, he spent almost half an hour with me. He never glanced at the clock. He was both professional and friendly. He smiled and made eye contact. Except for my physical exam, he remained seated and clearly answered all my questions. It reminded me how important communication is for physicians. It must be challenging to read a patient when they first meet them to figure out how to talk to them like they aren't stupid, but in a way they understand. Translating recurrence rates, statistics and risk factors into layperson terms takes talent and skill.

He wasn't rushed and didn't seem to be trying to wrap the appointment up in any way. I never felt as if I was intruding on his time. He was there for me for the entire 30 minutes. He said a number of times, "If you ever want to come back and see us, just give us a call." He shook my hand again when he got up to leave.

I walked back to my car feeling calm and relaxed. I felt as if I was taken care of, mostly because of how this young physician behaved and not what he did. His friendly, calm, unrushed manner turned what could have been a stressful and upsetting oncology appointment into a perfectly fine oncology appointment.

I assert that the so-called bedside manner matters a lot. While our interaction might have been just an ordinary appointment, it meant much more than that to me. I've said it before but it bears repeating: it is these little things – a handshake, a smile, patience, eye contact, a calm manner – that mean a lot to us vulnerable, broken patients, every single time.

Medicine might cure (sometimes), it doesn't always heal. This oncologist was not only a specialist, smart and brimming with lots of medical knowledge, but he was a healer too. And right then, I mostly needed to heal.

Cheers to all the healers out there, who comfort and alleviate suffering just by holding space for their patients. Holding space is the ultimate demonstration of respect for patients. I strongly believe that it is these gentle folks who will help us heal in the end.

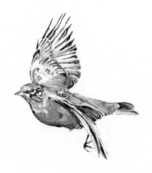

Reflections

The Bedrock
of Health Care

∽ what patient centred care means to me ∽

We are all just walking each other home.

– Ram Dass

ll my stories dance on the edges of patient centred care. I
fear that patient centred care is a term used so often that it
has become meaningless jargon. The phrase is slapped on hospital
strategies at an alarming rate. I contend that you can't say you are
patient centred until patients say you are patient centred.

Patient centred care has birthed other phrases like patient experience and patient engagement. Now my head is swimming with all
these corporate terms.

I'd say that my experiences in health care are stories that illustrate
the foundational elements of patient centred care: respect, dignity,
information sharing and collaboration.

These foundations can apply to any relationship in health care. To
be healthy in the health care system, we all need these elements –
patients, families, staff and physicians.

Respect is what underpins all relationships. Trust is built on a bedrock of respect. But respect is such a vague term. What does respect look like in a health care setting?

This is what respect looks like to me as a patient: respect is knocking at the door before entering. It is asking, "Is this a good time to come in?" It is introducing yourself, along with your role and what you are there to do. It is engaging in chitchat to get to know each as human beings, not just as patients and professionals. It is slowing down and even sitting down if you can. It is not appearing rushed if you are rushed. It is making eye contact. It is smiling.

It is asking the patient what they like to be called. It is not calling a mom Mom or a child Buddy. It is using proper names.

It is pausing for an answer after you ask a question. It is not interrupting. It is saying, "What questions do you have?", and then waiting, instead of the often-rushed "Do you have any questions?", asked as you are heading out the door. Respect helps us build trust and we cannot have a healthy relationship with someone we don't trust.

My old friend dignity is mostly about privacy. This means allowing our bodies as much dignity as possible. This means minimizing the flapping patient gowns – the paper gowns are the worst. It also means at least offering a gown so we don't experience undue nudity. Covering someone up as you examine them. Finding a private room to have conversations. Not speaking about patients at reception, in elevators or other public places.

Information sharing is much more than handing a patient a pamphlet. When I waited for my cancer surgery, many people gave me pamphlets. I politely accepted them and shoved them in a file folder when I got home. I did not read a single pamphlet.

Just because you give someone a pamphlet doesn't mean you've shared information with them.

Health literacy is the responsibility of health professionals, not patients. If people have low health literacy, it just means the professionals have not explained things in a way that people can understand. This includes offering information that has been translated for language and culture – which so rarely happens in health care. Almost all the patient education materials are in English, not in plain language or with accessible graphic design, and created with the assumption that people can read. That leaves many people behind in the dust.

Collaboration is the final cornerstone of good health care. This is the most challenging part of the equation because health care is rife with power imbalances. It is impossible to collaborate if you have no power. In order for patients to acquire power, health care has to give up some of its own power.

In my experience, authentic collaboration is rare. People and systems are reluctant to hand over any power. I'll illustrate this point with a story.

Once my son went to the audiologist to get his hearing tested. The appointment started off well, with me smiling and extending my hand so the audiologist could shake it. But then I made a crucial mistake: I started asking questions. We had waited months for the appointment and I had many questions. First, I asked about why there weren't sound systems installed in the schools, musing that a sound system would benefit my son.

"You don't have to tell me what a sound system is," the audiologist snapped, asserting her power as an expert over me.

I took a deep breath and said to her, "Can you please speak to me more respectfully?"

The appointment went downhill from there. I did not do my job to be a compliant mother. I was not being a good caregiver. Good caregivers are expected to be quiet and passive.

In response, she directed Aaron into the soundproof room where they did the hearing testing and slammed the door behind them, leaving me sitting alone in the little wait area. I didn't know where they went, how long they would be, or what she was doing with my son. She walked in and out of the booth a few times, not acknowledging me at all as she adjusted levels for Aaron during his hearing test. I clearly had been a bad caregiver, and she made sure to punish me for that.

Now I sat back watching this whole experience unfold. I knew that Aaron was fine – although she spoke to him as if he was dumb as a post and about two years old, not 13. But she wasn't mean to him. I tried to focus on Aaron's experience instead and thought about the impression I made with her.

A mom comes in (me) and has a lot of questions about her son's hearing. Damnit, she's the expert, not this mom, so she needs to assert her power over me to put me in my place. It worked. Taking my son from me, not telling me what was happening, I felt shamed and small. She had won. From her perspective, I had questioned her expertise by asking questions. I'll admit I could have shown more reverence towards her. But I also believe strongly that it is okay for patients and families to ask questions.

Partnerships are built between two people who trust one another and acknowledge each other's expertise. Liking each other helps too, but liking each other isn't mandatory.

In this case, I was the expert in being my son's mom, and the audiologist was an expert in audiology. We should have come together because of what we had in common: concern for Aaron's hearing. We both became all prickly with each other, so there was no chance for collaboration.

Respect, dignity, information sharing and collaboration. It is pure magic when this happens in a health care encounter. Reflecting back on our son's first appointment with Dr. Darwish, his pediatrician, I know that every single moment can have these elements, so I know it can be done. When there's a will, there's a way.

Does the Spirit Catch You?

~ an examination of patient culture and health care culture ~

> **...instead of inquiring about the physician's skill**
> **or credentials, he asked, "Do you know someone**
> **who would care for me and love me?"**
> *– Anne Fadiman*

T his one stunning statement from Anne Fadiman's book, *The Spirit Catches You and You Fall Down*, embodies my entire philosophy about what is going terribly wrong with our health system.[1]

I devoured this book and began recommending it to my health care friends – some because they "got it" and it would validate their approach to caring for others, and others because they did not get it at all. I hoped for those who are philosophically misaligned with me that this book would be their epiphany to stop judging, eye rolling and labelling the patients and their families whose values were not the same as their own.

The Spirit Catches You and You Fall Down is a call for understanding and compassion. It is a simply told story about a very complex situation, which is no easy feat in writing. I have deep respect for writer

Anne Fadiman.

The Lees, a family of Hmong origin, arrive in California as refugees from Southeast Asia. They present at the local hospital with their young daughter named Lia, who is diagnosed with epilepsy. Great miscommunication between the family and the health providers ensues, and eventually Lia experiences brain damage. The family blames the doctors; the physicians blame the non-compliant parents. In the end, it is the family who is correct. Lia's well-meaning, highly educated physicians injure her with their woeful ignorance.

While some might classify this tale as a story of a child's acquired brain injury, this is really the story of a family's unconditional love. It shares cautionary lessons that reflect poorly on the rigid close-hearted health professionals. Blaming neither the family nor the system, it is the people who are Lia's health care providers who let this family down. The professionals neither care for nor love the family, and dismiss them as foreign, obstinate, non-compliant and plain stupid. This value-laden lens does not even begin to touch the complexities of this family and their culture. It is the highly educated ones who end up terribly wrong.

As Anne Fadiman says, "The Westerners' knowledge was not a gift. It was coercion." She says she stood in awe of Lia's parents, Foua and Nao Kao, who "stood firm in the face of expert opinion."

This book is so important on so many levels, and I'm heartened to hear it is required reading in some medical schools.

It calmly points out the great inequities of our Western health system, where it is demanded that parents surrender all control of their child when they walk through the hospital doors. The Hmong culture has no class system, which means that "nobody was more important than anybody else." This disregard of physicians' status infuriated most doctors, who were used to being at the top of their medical pecking order. This book also points out how people working in the health system immediately view difference as inferiority.

The only people who showed compassion towards the Lee family were the ones who paused to try to understand the why behind the family's actions. And if they could not understand the why, they chose to simply accept the family instead.

This is a book about cultural humanity. My most illuminating take-away is that medicine has its own very strong culture that demands compliance from its patients based purely on its own perceived superiority. But what if the so-called experts aren't the experts at all? What if it is patients and families who are the experts, and it is the professionals that are simply temporary lenders of knowledge?

There is a concluding passage that strikes me at a personal level, as it speaks to the value of difference.

While the health providers throw their hands up at Lia when she becomes permanently disabled, labelling her a "vegetable," the author disagrees.

"How can I say she is not valuable when she means to much to the people around her? How can I say she has nothing to contribute when she altered the course of my family life, my life as a writer and my whole way of thinking...?"

This is a transformational book. Maybe we've placed importance on all the wrong things – what if the solution to healing people is not knowledge and expertise – it is caring and love instead?

Notes

1. Fadiman, Anne, The Spirit Catches You and You Fall Down: A Hmong Child, Her American Doctors, and the Collisions of Two Cultures. 2012. https://www.amazon.ca/Spirit-Catches-You-Fall-Down/dp/0374533407

Why Is This
A Competition?

~ how there is ridiculous competition ~
between different diagnoses

**The way to right wrongs is to turn
the light of truth upon them.**
– Ida B. Wells-Barnett

While I'm a newbie to the cancer world, I have been the
mom to a kid with a disability for 16 years. In both the
illness and disability communities, I have detected a weird under-
current of competition.

In the disability community this look like: whose kid is more
disabled and requires more care? Who has an invisible disability?
A visible one? Governments also love to make funding decisions
based on this competition. Bureaucrats decide who needs support,
respite or childcare, not families or disabled people.

Competing fractures our connections. In all this competition for
dollars, compassion and care has broken the disability community into a million tiny pieces based on diagnosis. As a result, our
fundraising, advocacy and support networks are all built sepa-
rately, in siloes. We are weaker as a community when we are torn

apart like this.

The best people rise above this competition. I love when I connect with a mom about what we have in common – how awesome our kids are as well as struggles with schools, health care, government funding and society. Families do not purely connect based on our kids' different diagnoses.

Aaron has a lot in common with kids with different disabilities. The same is true with cancer. I can connect with people who have had any type of cancer, not just breast cancer. I've also been blessed to meet many folks in the chronic disease world who have been kind and supportive to me. They don't have to have cancer to offer empathy on topics like body image, pain or identity. Together we are all stronger.

Cancer has a pecking order. Have lung cancer? Expect constant questions about if you smoked (and so what if you did?). Have skin cancer? Ditto the questions about tanning or sun exposure. Have any kind of cancer at all? Many remarks about your unhealthy lifestyle will be slung your way.

I consider this dumping on people who are the most vulnerable. This is the tiresome "blame the patient" phenomenon. Isn't just having cancer (or a baby with a disability) enough for a little bit of kindness? It feels like we are all competing for a finite amount of compassion in this messed-up world.

Dig deeper and breast cancer has its own weird order.

Mastectomy (single or double) or partial mastectomy. Chemotherapy or no chemotherapy. Radiation or no radiation. Estrogen blockers or not. I didn't have chemo and have felt that I don't fit into the traditional world of breast cancer. One nurse said to me, "Well, radiation isn't as bad as chemo." Which I'm sure is true, but because I didn't have chemo, radiation was the worst thing that happened to me. The first day I had radiation was one of the worst days of my life.

But I bite my tongue because I know there are others who have been through much more taxing treatment. This suppresses my own pain, which leaks out in other ways.

This moves into prognosis too. There is a difference in compassion and research funding between early stage cancer patients and those who have metastatic cancer, which is woefully ignored and underfunded.

Let's embrace each other without tearing each other down. Let's recognize that we have more in common than not and stop allowing governments, society and systems to fracture us apart.

As a wise person once told me, "You can't lose if you don't play the game." Choose to not compare. If we make it safe for every patient and caregiver (and health professional, too) to tell their stories, then all the things that separate us will magically disappear. We are all in this together.

Tattoo Me

~ my effort to take my body back from health care ~

Self-care: this might make things suck less.
– Megan Devine

As I get older, I have become an accumulation of scars. A hernia repair when I was eight years old left two faint, raised scars. I have three small scars on my forearms from testing for a bleeding disorder. Two attempts to remove an ovary resulted in a keloid scar in my belly button. My partial mastectomy left a one-inch scar that just peeks out of my bikini top. I have another scar and a hematoma that lingered for months under my arm from lymph node removal.

I understand the medical need for these scars. They are evidence of removing things that were causing me trouble. Along with scars, breast cancer gifted me with two permanent radiation tattoos.

I was at an appointment to prep for radiation. The radiation therapist took out this box thing with a needle and ink. And then she proceeded to poke me with it in two places – right in my cleavage and on the side of my ribcage. This was bizarre and these tattoos look like blackheads. I asked if she could at least make them into flowers but she didn't think that was funny.

They put stickers on me, too, and drew on me with a pen each radiation treatment. My boob looked like a piece of meat about to be butchered. At least the stickers and pen wore off. The tattoos were permanent.

I asked a friend who is a radiation therapist, "Why the need for permanent marks for radiation that is over in four weeks?" She told me there isn't a semi-permanent alternative.

This falls into the category of: what is a big deal for me isn't a big deal for health care professionals. What I didn't like was the permanent nature of something that the hospital only needs for a few weeks. This seems to tread on my dignity.

It strikes me that there are many side effects from procedures in the hospital that are crappy for patients, but convenient for clinicians so nobody does anything to change it.

My friend did add, "There is quite a bit of research looking at alternatives like henna, UV lighting and 'invisible' tattoos and external surface landmark light systems."

To this, I say, "Yes, yes please do more research." As a patient, this is important to me. I don't want a stupid blackhead tattoo looking at me for the rest of my life. If patients like me were engaged to set priorities in cancer research, I'd ask to figure out a way to get rid of the damn permanent tattoos, pronto.

Little black dots might seem minor in the grand scheme of things, but I didn't like losing even more control of my suffering body one little bit. Later, I asked my nice radiation oncologist if it was medically okay to get a tattoo on my breast to cover up my radiation tattoo.

He said very solemnly, "There are no counter-indications to getting a tattoo." He probably thought, "This woman is clearly in the midst of a mid-life crisis and losing her marbles", but he was too polite to express this judgment.

So, to reclaim my own damn body, I got my very own tattoo to cover up the radiation tattoo on my breast. I went to a place called Hula

Girl Tattoo. The young dudes working there have seen everything and they didn't even blink at my request. I told them they were doing good work to cover up a mom's cancer tattoo.

Part of getting my tattoo was to say, "Take that, health care system! I am in charge of what permanent marks adorn my body!" I wanted to send the cancer hospital the bill for the tattoo.

My new cover-up tattoo is a constellation of hearts with a sprinkling of stars. A purple star has replaced the ugly radiation tattoo. One of the hearts is for my husband Mike, who was my unwavering support. The other heart is for me, to remind me to love myself.

It hurt to get the tattoo, especially the part near my sternum, but Mike was there to hold my hand, exactly as he did during the whole cancer saga. Tears leaked out of my eyes, not because of the pain, but because I felt grateful my treatment was done, my cancer was caught early and I'm alive to tell the tale.

My new tattoo is a symbol of my own story of having cancer. This is my story to tell, not cancer's. Slowly, slowly, I started taking my power back, one heart in my constellation at a time.

SUE ROBINS

Our Sisterhood
of Pain

$\sim$ the pressure to present as a good patient $\backsim$

It is not our differences that divide us.
It is our inability to recognize, accept,
and celebrate those differences.
– Audre Lorde

I brought my red Moleskine notebook to every oncologist appointment. In it I carefully recorded the date and the questions
I needed answered. I hadn't seen my official oncologist in months. I
caught a glimpse of her in the staff room and hallway, but she didn't
see me. Instead, I got the family physician in the clinic or the oncologist resident. I know this is how it works. I'm post-treatment with a
boring low-grade cancer – and I don't want to be an interesting case
for an oncologist – but I can't help but feel unimportant because of
this rejection.

Today, regardless of who I see, I try to be organized and look put
together for whoever shows up in the treatment room. If I'm feeling
stronger and in self-advocating mode, I'm sure to dress up and have
makeup on. Is it wrong of me to do this, to lean on my privilege? I've

learned over the years that I get listened to and taken seriously by clinicians if I look and act like them as much as possible.

I once heard of a mom who was an Indigenous woman who had a kid with a disability. Every time she went to the children's hospital, she dressed up in a (goddamn) business suit to purposely over-compensate for the shocking power inequities between patients/families and health care professionals. This power imbalance was exacerbated by the fact she was Indigenous. Is this okay? No. No, it is not okay.

The worst part is that sometimes health professionals don't even realize they contribute to these imbalances with their obliviousness to their own privilege.

I don't need someone to give me a voice. I already have a voice. I need someone to listen. If I have to get dressed up to be heard, I get dressed up. Should I be able to present disheveled in my sweatpants? I should, but then I'll be judged. This isn't paranoia; it is my reality.

I've been written off as a "hysterical mom" many times when I've accompanied my son to the clinic or hospital. I'm careful not to show emotion – to not cry or to raise my voice, even if I'm upset. As a patient or family member, I wish to be treated by health profession-als with the same common courtesy that is afforded to a colleague.

Think of me as someone you love, then, if that helps. As your sister, wife or mom. No matter how well-dressed or well-spoken (or not) I am.

Recently, there was yet another article published in a medical journal written by a physician who became a patient. I appreciate the author's humbleness and recognition of his own privilege. Here is a male oncologist/patient, asking for the receptionist to smile. I've been calling for receptionists to smile for years, but who am I? I am just another layperson patient, a middle-aged breast cancer patient, a mom of a kid with Down syndrome. I do not have an oncologist's platform. Health care loves to listen to doctors. To regular people, not so much. Therein lies the problem.

It is important to note that I am white, reasonably well-off economically, generally well-spoken and I have worked in health care administration my entire career – specifically in patient and family experience for the past 13 years. Alas, I am also a woman and a patient, which knocks me down a few rungs on the health care ladder of status. I struggle to be taken seriously.

There are starting to be stories about how much of this power imbalance is due to gender. I applaud these stories. May they continue to be told.

A Collage of Hope

～ the healing power of art ⌒

If your heart is broken, make art with the little pieces.

– Shane Koyczan

W alking the cluttered halls of the cancer hospital as a patient, I saw very little that was welcoming or patient-friendly. Pictures were crammed into displays on the walls. There were some pieces that were donated by a family of a patient who had died, like a large lovely quilt. This is a nice sentiment, but it is also disconcerting for the patients who were still alive and roaming the halls.

I had a burning desire to do something with my radiation treatment photos. I had taken one photo for each day I had radiation, twenty in all.

Lining the walls of the cancer hospital were photographs. They were not photographs from patients, however – they were the results of a staff photography contest. Could there really be anything more provider centred than the results of a photography contest for staff lining the hospital walls? Physical space does speak to the culture of an organization.

"Wouldn't it be nice to have patient photos on the walls?" silly me thought. I asked this question to the patient experience person.

Here is her response:

> *"We no longer have the ability at the cancer hospital to share*
> *individual patient stories...as the policy at the hospital restricts*
> *us from privileging one story over another."*

I sat on that response for a long time and never responded. Her answer was no, no, no. After I read it, I felt shame flood my face for even asking. If a patient experience person can't be kind, or invite ideas from patients – well, the whole organization is hopeless.

Instead, she suggested I come to their focus group instead (already scheduled, the next week, at a time I have to pick my kid up from school). I did not attend. This is not the way you engage. This is the way you disengage.

My photos sat on my private Instagram account, unused for many months. I wanted to do something with them, but I didn't know what. It dawned on me that creating art with them would be a way to bring closure to that difficult time in my life.

I have a friend who is a visual artist. She also happens to be living with a chronic disease. We had met a couple of times for coffee and to connect by both railing against and laughing at the absurdities of health care.

One day, she generously invited me over to her apartment to teach me how to create a collage with my photos. I had sat with the pictures for many months and realized that they were not silly photos; they were a symbol of my pain from that dark time last year. I had a need to communicate them, to craft them into some sort of story. The patient experience person did not understand that, but my friend did.

I arrived at her place bearing raisin and oatmeal cookies and photocopies of my pictures. She had also asked me to collect images from magazines. She had all the supplies to collage. I was fortunate enough to stumble upon a talented friend who had also taught collage classes when her health permitted.

Her white-whiskered black lab greeted me at the door. I sat at her kitchen table, happily cutting, pasting, drinking tea and munching on cookies for the entire morning.

There was something soothing about the whole process of creating my little collage. I layered image upon image, my black and white pictures of radiation peeking out amongst more joyful photos of my children and polka-dotted stencils. I added birds and a piece of measuring tape. The collage was a picture of that time – a combination of dark images – like the long hospital hall, a selfie in a changing room mirror, my husband on a waiting room chair. In the corner were colour photos of my children and their spouses, who were really my shining light during my cancer treatment. I struggled hard with feeling worthless and devalued. My loved ones were, some days, the only reason I even bothered to show up for radiation appointments. In the dark, I had a sliver of light.

These are images from a time I'd rather forget. But those twenty days are etched so deeply inside of me that my only way out is to weave that time into my very being. Creating a visual story through a collage worked for me. I am forever grateful to my artist friend for dedicating a day to me.

This is why telling our stories – in whatever form – is so important. By gathering our experience into a story, we make sense of random or traumatic events. It is only then that we begin to heal. I look at my completed collage with both sorrow and fondness.

The Patient Storyteller

~ allowing the space for patients to tell their stories ~

**Have compassion for me for being vulnerable enough
to tell my story. Even if you are uncomfortable.**

– Morgan Jerkins

My own writing in the early days after my cancer diagnosis was a hot mess, reflective of the chaos I was experiencing in real-time in my life. My journal entries two weeks after my partial mastectomy surgery are particularly painful.

March 3, 2017

I'm circling the drain here.

*Have a terrible awful huge swollen spot under my incision. A seroma?
A hematoma? Not sure. Went to family doctor today and am grateful to
be on antibiotics and more pain killers. Terrified it is going to burst or get
infected and I'm going to end up in emergency. Or with sepsis. I think this
is awfully big. Have to wait to see surgeon. I see how this health stuff is all
consuming.*

Mostly in pain – just furrowed brow stuff and can think of nothing else. In desperation, I sent Mike out to the grocery store 10 minutes before closing to buy a whole cabbage. Remembering my La Leche Leader days, we pull off the inner leaves to apply to my swollen spot. This helps women with engorged breasts. Maybe it will help me. Silly but seems harmless.

I eat oranges cut into eight slices every night after dinner in my bed. I watch Say Yes to the Dress endlessly. Aaron and I watch our recorded cooking shows: MasterChef, Top Chef. He tells me he wants to go to Toronto and be the first Down syndrome chef on MasterChef. I nod and agree – that would be great.

Earlier in the day, he said, "Mom, stop being like an animal." "An animal?" I say, confused. "Yes, a monkey" – and then he jumped around like a monkey. I can see why he thinks I'm like a monkey with my endless tidying up and puttering. You should be more like a human being, he decided. I agree.

My family doctor said today, "Try not to worry" and gave me a hug. Ella tells me not to worry too. I am worried. Now I'm worried I'm going to get a blood infection and die of sepsis. Mike and I decide our plan if I quickly deteriorate: call the ambulance. Follow me to the hospital afterwards with Aaron. Mike can try to find a babysitter when they are there. I'm keen not to upset Aaron too much. Maybe when our neighbours return from Mexico, they can be our emergency back-up plan.

I keep reading breast cancer blogs but many of the women who have written the blogs have died or they have metastatic cancer. This scares me. I wish it didn't scare me. Many Twitter feeds haven't been updated in years. I know what that means. The women behind the Twitter accounts are gone.

I tried all sorts of storytelling to write my way through my cancer. I wrote in my journal. I handwrote in the variety of little notebooks that I carried around with me. I typed out thoughts on my phone. I texted myself. I crafted stories to make sense of things and those I posted on my blog. I signed up for a poetry class, where all I wrote about was cancer and memories of my beloved grandmother.

Writing made me feel a wee bit better. Sometimes I just wrote in my private journal and sometimes I posted on my blog. An extended family member told me, "Your blog is too difficult for me to read." I smiled and nodded. Was I to write things to make her feel better?

"Well then don't read it then," I thought in my head, hurt by her criticism. I know now that I was trying to sort out my own chaos through my writing. This was a good thing, not a bad thing.

Life's chaotic interruptions are what shape us. Loss, loss and more loss are the hallmarks of life. Nobody is guaranteed a pain-free life. It is a sad day indeed when we cannot express our own sorrow in whatever way makes the most sense for us.

What stories can do is neutralize our chaos, but we need time and space to tell them. Health care is reluctant to entertain true patient stories. Authentic patient stories interfere with the system's preferred narrative, which is what Arthur Frank terms as restitution.[1]

A restitution story sounds like "I was sick, the hospital cured me and now life is better than ever!" Tack onto this restitution narrative is the fact that clinicians are trained as heroes who always save the day. If our days are not saved, then they are no longer heroes. People don't want to hear the failed hero story. The only failed hero of this story of restitution is me, the patient.

Hospitals expect sick people to get well and to never talk about the actual visceral, traumatic experience of being ill. This is medicine's obsession with their own curative model. This happens a lot in the cancer world, where a chase for the cure is especially strong. In reality, there is no cure for cancer.

The way out of the chaotic storm of illness is to tell stories. The best sort of people are those who create space for stories. They can sit with an uncomfortable story without minimizing it, interrupt-

ing, looking for the bright side, correcting the storyteller or running away. Encouraging patients to tell their own stories in their
own way paves the road towards healing.

Notes
1. Frank, Arthur, The Wounded Storyteller, 1995, https://www.press.uchicago.edu/ucp/books/
book/chicago/W/bo14674212.html

We All Have
Our Own Stories

~ how patients are much more than their data ~

Maybe stories are just data with a soul.

– Brené Brown

Medicine collects the technical aspects of the illness story, not the emotional parts of the story. I quickly found out if you start wandering into the land of feelings, you will get referred to a psychiatrist.

The data associated with my illness offers up little meaning to my illness. People – even people who work in health care – find stories of patient experiences in crisis upsetting because it conflicts with the concept of health care curing and living happily ever after.

I once heard a radiation therapist say, "Well, patients are always upset when they start radiation but then they get used to it."

This statement speaks to many things: The dismissing of the initial emotion, the idea that being upset at the beginning doesn't matter because we get used to it. Just because we've gotten used to it and cease to show emotions halfway through our regime of radiation doesn't mean that lying beneath a huge radiation machine that's pumping poison into our bodies doesn't cause pain and trauma to both our physical and mental selves.

I wonder if this is a protective mechanism. This attitude dismissing an element of a cancer experience might make the person who is responsible for administering the radiation feel better about their job.

"At least you didn't need chemo. Radiation is not so bad." I heard this many times.

Perhaps instead of opening up their hearts to nurture compassion for the suffering patient, some clinicians have shut down and become dismissive so they don't have to recognize their role in inflicting pain. Maybe they don't want to visit the pain that may be in themselves, so they pretend that there's no suffering at all. I don't know. I do know that I think it would be better if we were all more honest with each other.

Stories signal our willingness to tell the truth about an experience. Our stories about the exact same experiences can be wildly different, depending on our perspective.

I notice this as a caregiver to Aaron. I often say, "We have a pediatrician" – not "Aaron has a pediatrician." His pediatrician feels like my doctor too, especially when Aaron was smaller and I did all the talking for him. Now that he's older, I realize that his doctor is his doctor and that his story is his story – not mine.

We are working towards Aaron using his own voice with his physician. Often, I will come in at the beginning of his medical appointment, say what's important to me, and then leave to have Aaron speak to his doctor alone. I have no idea what goes on in those conversations – sometimes Aaron shows up with a prescription, but often he leaves the clinic room with simply a wave to his physician. I am not briefed afterwards and I know this is as it should be.

When I was in cancer treatment, my husband would say, "We are in treatment." I have to say, although I love this guy terribly, this annoyed me. I pointed out that I was the person lying under the radiation machine and sometimes he was in the waiting room and sometimes he was at work.

If I take the "you have your story and he has his story" philosophy, I can see now that my husband also has a cancer story. This is despite the fact that he did not have cancer. His story is parallel to mine, as my story is parallel to my son's story with Down syndrome. But they are all different stories.

The error I've made as Aaron's mother over the years is that I've assumed that my story is Aaron's story. Because I communicate faster than Aaron does, my story often trumped his story. This is not okay.

I've often heard disabled people speak up against their caregivers. They say it is horrible to hear that their mothers were distraught when they were born. It was awful to endure years of therapy to try to "fix" them to make them "normal" again – mostly for the family's sake. I can see that I've done this too and I hang my head in shame.

Sometimes the caregiver's story overshadows the story of the person who is actually the patient or the "subject" of the story. This could be because caregivers have a strong need to tell their stories too. I do not think we should squash caregivers' stories but they should not overshadow a patient story.

Stories can help heal people who work in health care too. We must all be careful of not co-opting other patient stories for our own benefit. Patient stories should be ideally told by the patients themselves. Taking the time to understand a diverse range of patient stories is important.

We need to make space for all stories. Patient stories, caregiver stories, staff and physician stories. We all have our own stories. There is healing in the telling of stories. Let's not deny anybody that.

Writing Your Way Through Cancer

∽ using poetry to process the cancer experience ∽

**Storytelling is less a work of reporting
and more a process of discovery.**

– Arthur Frank

My experiences as a patient were uncomfortable and that's what made my writing uncomfortable to read. The things that make us uncomfortable are also the things that make us grow. For health professionals, reading a variety of first-person accounts written by patients can help to nurture empathy towards those they care for.

April 12, 2017

A big mess of feeling dead inside, being really angry at other stuff (disability services stuff) and trying, trying, trying so hard. Doing a bit of work on the book. Meditating. Appreciating our view. Going for a walk. Doing nice things for myself.

My brain is less mush, more complete sentences, which is not necessarily a good thing.

I shouldn't be surprised by everybody who has forgotten about me. What a flood of cards, gifts and messages right after diagnosis and now nothing. Like after I'm diagnosed, it is over. Strange but not.

Still buying cancer books, but none have spoken to me. Have read a disproportionate amount by women with metastatic cancer. What if that doctor, who doesn't even know me, read my pathology wrong? What if she's just trying to save money by not giving me chemo and dismissing me? What if she's rationing care? I don't think I'm interesting to her. I didn't like her. I hope the radiation oncologist is better.

She said I would have to pay for the oncdx test. Why am I only stage 1, not stage 2a? My tumour seems big enough. Probably so they don't have to pay for the test. No genetic test either. I think they are skimping on me.

I am supposed to be knitting. I am paralyzed until I find out my FUCK-ING SCHEDULE. I bet I won't get it on Tuesday either. I will have to wait some more.

Yesterday I was flat. I slept the morning away. Dragged myself out of bed because the sun was shining and walked to the poké bar. Ate poké out on the terrace. That helped. (Although I put on my jeans today and should really cut back on the spicy mayo and ice cream and such).

I spent a lot of time in between appointments even before my treatment began. First I healed from surgery and then I waited. I kept ordering books online. They'd show up in my mailbox a few days later and I'd carefully stack them on the coffee table. I read and I walked.

I felt dead inside with all the waiting. I kept writing on my blog. In my private journal, I tried to process my feelings of being abandoned by people who I thought loved me. This abandonment brought more pain than I thought I could endure but writing helped alleviate this a little bit.

I became agitated and then depressed from spending too much

time alone in our condo during the day, especially when the West Coast rain came. I searched for other places to write that weren't noisy coffee shops.

One day I wandered over to our local arts centre. It was perched on the shores of a lake, all rolling hills and shady trees. There were tables inside of the hushed space which was filled with art and studios. It seemed like a good place to set up my laptop.

I kept returning to that peaceful space. One day I picked up a program about classes. There was a session called Writing in the Morning that was offered at 10 a.m. every second Monday morning. Impulsively I signed up. I needed some form of structure for my days. I had bi-weekly therapy appointments that kept me going, but I'd often look at my date book on a Sunday night and realize it was totally devoid of plans. At least I'd have a writing class twice a month.

Surprising to me, it was at this new class where I started to write poems.

I see now:
I was writing my way out of my cancer.
Gathering the courage to speak.
Telling my truth through fiction.
And slowly taking up my rightful space again.

I arrived at my first class with no expectations. I assumed we'd have three hours to write in our journals. I had no idea that it was actually a poetry workshopping class. Our instructor would read to us, give us a prompt, we'd have time to write a poem and then read it out loud in the class. I had never written poetry and I had cancelled all my public speaking engagements to avoid speaking in front of people about my pain. This workshopping idea terrified me. If I had known this was the format for this class, I would have never signed up.

It was not too bad. Everybody had to read their poems, so I did not feel alone. The instructor was kind and not critical.

I ended up remaining at the class for six months. It seemed to have a place and time in my recovery. I am not a good poet. I am rambling and unable to incorporate the nature metaphors that seemed popular in the class. I wrote literal poems which were just chopped up versions of my prose. I did meet another mom in the class who had just finished cancer treatment too. We started to meet each other outside of the class for coffee. I realized how much writing about our cancer contributed to feeling just a wee bit better.

I think about how a writing class supported by the cancer hospital would be a simple, yet profound offering for patients. Encouraging patients to share their stories would be one way to transform a cancer hospital from an impersonal medical treatment centre to a place for healing. Leaning on humanities of all sorts – writing, visual arts, music, movement – has so much untapped potential in the health care world.

The Best Solutions are Human Solutions

a commentary on how technology
should be a complement to care

Technology powered by love can save the world.

– Jane Chen

T echnology solutions in health care are hot right now. There's an
app for this and a website for that. But technology itself will not
save us; it is the human beings who will save health care.

I am married to an IT guy. He loves data, metadata, apps that give
him data, spreadsheets and numbers in general. When I was in labour with Aaron, my water had broken so the nurses hooked me up to
a fetal monitoring machine to gather data about my contractions. My
dear husband sat with his back to me, hypnotized by the fetal monitoring machine and all its glorious numbers, lights and beeping.

Mike announced every few minutes, "Sue, there is a contraction
coming!"

Unmedicated me yelled back at him, "I know there is a contraction coming! I can feel it!" The lights and numbers on the machine
had enticed him so much that he had forgotten about the real
person right beside him. I did not have a problem sternly reminding

him about the people part of health care, as he is my husband. I do have a tougher time speaking up to health professionals when I am in vulnerable health situations.

Being connected to that damn machine also meant I could not walk around because I was detained flat on my back. Technology interfered with allowing my body to do what it needed to do to get labour going.

After some data had been collected, I begged the nurses to unhook me from the machine. I was desperate to walk around to get labour going naturally, through the proven method of labouring women pacing the hospital hallways. I knew if I didn't walk around, I'd eventually get hooked up to a medication to induce me, which would in turn cause a bunch more interventions. I did not want that.

I was finally freed from the machine so I could walk about. Walking worked, and soon afterwards, my son was born.

Numbers, lights and beeping can mesmerize health professionals too. I wish there was as much attention and funding given to interpersonal relationships in health care as there is to technology. I think that technology should serve as a support, not a hindrance, to relationships.

It distresses me to have a computer screen between me and my doctor. It can be a barrier to interpersonal care. I know that electronic medical records can also be time-consuming for clinicians. This time would be better spent invested in face-to-face interactions with patients.

A few years after Aaron was born, I attended a Hacking Health event. Hacking Health is where people from diverse groups are brought together to work on innovate solutions to health care problems. Most of the solutions created at Hacking Health events are based in technology and digital health.

As the mom of a disabled kid, I pitched the problem of wayfinding to the audience of students, clinicians, technology people and designers. My wayfinding problem was a simple one. It was about Aaron and me getting lost in the hospital. I had only a minute to share my pitch in front of a packed auditorium. The fact I survived this brief but stressful speaking engagement was itself a miracle.

A Wayfinding Team took up my cause. They ended up winning a Hacking Health Award for innovation after two days of intensive design work. Their proposal was not a shiny new app to help patients navigate the hospital corridors, but for a people-powered solution instead. Their answer was to engage hospital volunteers to escort patients to their destinations in the hospital. This was true universal design in action, for more patients would be served by a real person taking them to their appointments than they would through a downloaded app.

In essence, the Wayfinding Team hacked Hacking Health with a human solution at a technology event. I believe that building a human solution is often much harder than building an app. While the relationship part of health care is sometimes dismissed by calling it soft, the soft stuff is what matters to me. Health care is about my relationship between me and my clinician, not me and my data.

How many applications are created by researchers and then never used by patients or families? While email and social media should serve as another way to communicate and connect people together, do we really need another app? Or, as the Hacking Health team showed us, do we instead need a real live person to show us the way? Technology can help but it is not the only solution to what ails us.

The Good Doctor

∽ an examination of the stress of medical appointments ⌒

Human knowledge is never contained in one person.
It grows from the relationships we create between each other
and the world, and still it is never complete.

– Paul Kalanithi

There is a prescribed amount of dread that comes along with having an appointment with the oncologist. I wonder if the people who work at the oncology clinic know this fact. I'm a train wreck by the time I show up to the reception desk.

So many patients are stumbling around the corridors with medical post-traumatic stress disorder (PTSD), a condition that can be avoided. This dread and additional trauma can dissipate with a positive experience or grow with a negative experience.

May 22, 2017

I had my oncology appointment last Thursday. I approached the day with my regular oncology dread.

Waking up at 5 a.m. with my head whirling; choosing my clothes carefully so I look somewhat credible (why do I have to do this to be taken seriously?); preparing my questions in my little notebook; driving white-knuckled to the appointment; listening to loud music – the Tragically Hip – in the car;

avoiding parking at the cancer hospital (the parkade there sends me into
a tailspin); getting there early so I can go for a walk beforehand; taking an
Ativan to calm the hell down (an Ativan prescribed to me by an oncologist –
that I only take when I have a health care appointment #irony); picking up
a coffee to bring with me to the clinic as a crutch/my armour; walking in like
my friend Isabel taught me, like I am The Queen; and asking the medical
assistant not to tell me how much I weigh (the very first thing they do there
is weigh me, my least favourite activity on earth). By the time the doctor
comes in, I am exhausted by my efforts to calm down.

Despite my many strategies to stay strong, I still sat in the windowless, joyless clinic room, waiting for a knock on the door, feeling
small, hunched over and nervously picking at my fingers until my
hangnails bled.

In the end, the person who knocked at the door was a senior
oncology resident. He was a pleasant man who forgot to introduce
himself, but he was otherwise lovely. I wish he had introduced himself because I was so nervous that I forgot to ask his name. He knew
my name but I did not know his, which caused a strange imbalance
to begin our relationship.

Introductions aside, what mattered to me is that we had an actual
conversation about the four questions I had written in my notebook.
Ours was a true back-and-forth exchange. I asked my questions and
he did not interrupt me while I was talking. He shared information
and options. He hesitated before he shared a thoughtful response.
He did not talk too fast. I listened and wrote in my little book and
then we discussed resolutions. I felt as if we tackled all my questions
together in a most collaborative way. This is called shared decision
making, but I mostly just call it respect. I felt seen by him as a real
person with important questions, not as a bothersome cancer patient who was taking up too much of his time. My dread had disappeared by the end of the appointment.

I left this interaction feeling greatly relieved. If this doctor thought I was hysterical or difficult, he didn't show it. If he was rushed or having a bad day, I didn't know. I appreciated his careful listening and consideration. It was a good experience with a good doctor. I felt hopeful that this young resident represented a new generation of physicians.

It saddens me that this ordinary appointment was extraordinary. A positive patient experience has been rare since I was diagnosed with cancer. This senior oncology resident treated me with courtesy and compassion. I felt validated, understood and listened to. His approach wasn't rocket science. I felt cared for by the way he treated me with simple respect.

This is how I wish all health care interactions should be, no matter one's gender, gender identity, ethnicity, citizenship, religion, race, disability, orientation, dress or eloquence.

It is humanity we all so crave from the health care system – no matter – or maybe because of – our different expressions of human identity. We are all people first. Doctors are people first and patients are people first too. The coming together in the realization of this shared humanity is really the foundation of health care.

Everybody is a Health Professional

the importance of every single
person who works in health care

**Could a greater miracle take place than for us to
look through each other's eyes for an instant?**
– Henry David Thoreau

Everybody who works in a hospital should consider themselves
a health professional. Every single staff member is paid to care
for patients, whether directly or indirectly. This includes the trades-
person who works in the physical plant, the clerks in health records
and the staff in food services.

There is a lady who works as a cashier in the cafeteria, which is in
the basement of a local hospital. I sometimes go to the cafeteria to
buy a coffee just to see her.

She is delighted to see every single customer, both staff and patients. Recently she exclaimed, "What a pretty necklace!" to me – I
blushed and put my hand to my neck, fingering the jewels on it. She
finds something positive to say to every single person who comes
through her lineup. She brightens up everybody's day.

It is fair to say that every single person in a hospital, including the

staff, could use some day-brightening. This woman is not a clinician, and in fact, she doesn't even work for the hospital, as she is
employed by the outsourced catering company. But she has realized
something: it is within her control to make people feel just a little bit
better – simply by her kind words and actions. Health care environments should be about making people feel better.

Most reception desks are built to be high up, with the receptionist towering over the patient (worse if you are a child or you use a
wheelchair). There is such value in a smile and eye contact when
a patient walks up to a desk. Expressing a welcome, or thanks for
coming is a nice way to start a conversation. It helps to use the
patient's name, and to explain why you are asking for information,
like address and health care card number.

When my appointments started up, I parked in the hospital
parkade. There were two ladies who staffed the parking booth. In
my dozens of visits, neither of them ever made eye contact with me
when I pulled up to pay my $15 fee. "Hello!" I chirped, desperate for
a smile or some attention, but they would walk through the whole
transaction without meeting my gaze or saying anything at all.
"Thank you so much!" I'd say before I drove off. Still nothing. It became a little game for me to see if I could get either of them to smile.
I never succeeded.

The parkade was a missed opportunity for simple kindness. The
attendants had the ability to brighten someone's day with a smile.
Perhaps these ladies had become jaded from months of seeing suffering people approaching their booth. Perhaps they did not understand the concept of customer service. Perhaps they did not realize
the power that they owned, despite their title and wage. Maybe they
feared that cancer was contagious, like so many other people. Maybe
they were always having a bad day. Perhaps they too were suffering
in some way. I couldn't figure out why they never smiled.

Every single person who works in health care is part of the care. Care can be delivered by booking clerks, parking staff, security or receptionists simply by the way that they treat patients. Every interaction in health care is a choice: treat someone with kindness to demonstrate that you care about them – or don't.

The morgue in the children's hospital is in the basement, which is level L on the elevator buttons. It is housed underground along with the pharmacy, the parking office and maintenance. There is one security guard per shift assigned to oversee the morgue.

Bodies are brought down by hospital porters and taken away by funeral home staff. These are bodies of tiny babies born early or teenagers who have died in car accidents. Families sometimes go into the morgue. The security guard unlocks the door to let them in and stands silently by as they view their beloved child's body. Then the security guard escorts the family out to the elevator after all is done. He or she returns to their watch at the morgue door until the entire process inevitably happens again.

Security guards assigned to the morgue are not trained health care professionals. They are often employed by an agency and are not even employees of the hospital. They bear witness to the single most horrific time in a family's life without any preparation or debriefing. There are no staff meetings or reflective practice seminars for them. What they see is stunningly traumatic, and nobody in the hospital even gives them a second glance.

Once you open yourself up to different perspectives in the hospital, it transcends beyond the patient and their family. People have their own reasons for working in health care. The receptionist could choose to work in an accounting office, but instead she's in the cancer clinic. I have an inkling that everybody in health care, not only doctors and nurses, have their own reasons for working there. If you acknowledge that every single staff, physician and volunteer in

235

the hospital makes a difference in the experience of a patient, then everybody deserve to be treated with respect.

I Am a Patient and I Have Had an Experience

 ∽ a plea to not be afraid of constructive patient feedback ⌒

I don't think anyone can grow unless he's loved exactly as he is now,
appreciated for what he is rather than what he will be.

– Fred Rogers

I became even more of a pain in the ass when I got cancer.

My treatment is over now and I am running out of excuses for naps, begging off obligations and eating almond croissants. I am achingly exhausted earlier and earlier every day and I have been told this fatigue will continue for several weeks. This cancer treatment is killing my social life.

As my oncologist said, two minutes of radiation is like spending the day in the hot sun, so I lurched around during radiation with a version of constant sunstroke. My boob was super itchy which was an annoyance but not debilitating. I asked the radiation therapists, "Why do some people get burned and itchy, and some do not?" and they did not know. I have no idea what research is going on over at that fancy research building across the street, but apparently it is not research on side effects like itchy boobs.

I promised not to complain about my cancer, because I did not need chemo and I did not need a full mastectomy and for those reasons, I am lucky. My experience having breast cancer has been surprisingly complicated and not all pink ribbons and teddy bears. It shook me to my core.

I received a voicemail message from a manager at the cancer hospital. Apparently someone had forwarded a story on my blog and told him to call me to talk about my experience. I arranged to meet with him, so Mike and I showed up to his windowless office before one of my daily radiation treatments.

He was a pleasant fellow, new to his job. It was clear I had been labeled a complainer, when in fact I had not contacted them with a complaint at all. I was only writing about my own personal experience for my own blog. True, my blog is public, but it feels creepy that my blog was being monitored in this way. I felt reported. We chatted about the patient experience in general and I emphasized that I hadn't complained, but that I did have some ideas for improvement. He wrote down a few things and that was that.

Feeling discouraged, I then followed up, asking to meet with the administrator in charge of Patient Experience. I am a Patient and I have had an Experience after all. I never heard back from him. I can take a hint.

As I told the manager, I want to help. Patients have good ideas. But I do not have any credibility at this cancer place beyond being only a patient. To administrators, patients are a generic cluster of diagnoses, not real people with ideas or opinions. We are all a bunch of nobodies.

It was silly, or maybe arrogant, for me to think they want my help. When feedback from patients is solicited by hospitals, through tools like surveys and comment cards, it is okay. But when patients approach them with feedback that is not overtly asked for, we are shut down, brushed aside, minimized, gotten rid of, seen as a problem that needs to be handled. I see this now. We are supposed to shut up and be grateful for care. Me and my cancer boob will zip it for now and stop rabble-rousing with the organization (and please know that I am grateful for the care, and brought in nice chocolates for the radiation therapists to my last appointment) and move forward.

Maybe one day an authentic chance to give feedback will be offered to me. I was given a patient satisfaction survey to fill out on my last day of treatment, but it had only a tiny spot to write "one or two ideas for improvement." I dutifully scribbled in a couple of thoughts – about orientation and waiting rooms. I actually had about 100 ideas for improvement, but there was no room for them on the page. No matter.

Signs Signs Signs

∽ how physical space can welcome or agitate patients ∾

Sign, sign, everywhere a sign
Blockin' out the scenery, breakin' my mind.
– Five Man Electrical Band

"Violence, foul language and abusive behaviours are not acceptable" reads the sign that is taped to the reception desk in a clinic that offers child immunizations. This looks like a sign that you might see in prison.

I think to myself, "Perhaps if the environment was welcoming, families would be more inclined to get their children immunized?"

I know that patients do abuse staff and that's not okay. But is a sign really going to stop someone? What percentage of patients are actually abusive to staff? Does that one percent warrant the need for the other 99 percent to be treated like potential criminals?

If you must put up a sign about abusive behaviour, why not say instead, "We want to foster a culture of respect towards everybody." Emphasize the behaviour you want to see, not the behaviour you don't.

I count 28 different signs in an x-ray clinic's waiting room. Twenty-eight. Most of the signs say, "No cell phones!" I look around and all the patients in the waiting room are immersed in their cell phones. Clearly the multitude of signs is not working. It is 2019. Why no cell phones? Do they mean no talking on your cell phone? I'm befuddled by the time I'm finally called in for my x-ray.

There's another sign – this one a stop sign – at all the entrances in the hospital to remind people to wash their hands. This is the first impression that patients see right when they walk into the hospital. Stop, not welcome.

I know hand hygiene is important. I know that keeping staff safe from abuse is important. I can see how one might want to discourage patients from loudly talking on their cell phones. Although the receptionist is loudly talking on her phone and everyone sitting in the waiting room can hear details about a patient's name, birthdate and health condition. I'm confused by this double standard.

The majority of patients arrive in health care settings in some sort of distress. Why not first welcome them into the clinic or hospital? Why not install signs that say the word welcome in many different languages to create a positive first impression?

I contend that first impressions matter. They set the tone for the rest of the interaction. The physical space of a waiting room seems like a fairly easy thing to change so it is more patient-friendly.

Once I toured a children's hospital waiting rooms with a mom who had a daughter who used a wheelchair. We walked into a clinic that had chairs lined up against the walls.

"Where is my daughter supposed to sit?" the mom rightly said. There was no room for a wheelchair or other mobility device like a walker. The child's wheelchair would be blocking the aisle. This was not a welcoming environment for this young patient and her family.

There are ways to fix these physical problems and they have to do with universal design. This means designing waiting rooms so they work for everybody. Talking to patients and families about their ideas to improve waiting rooms would be a great first step. We probably have some good solutions because we spend a lot of time waiting in waiting rooms.

Waiting room environments could be healing environments. Replacing the tattered signs taped up on the wall with artwork would be a good start. Consider playing soft music to create a more peaceful setting. These are simple changes that can make a big difference.

A pre-admission clinic at a children's hospital has volunteers who sit on the floor and play with toys with young patients and their brothers and sisters while they wait for their appointments. This is a thoughtful gesture and both amuses the kids and allows the families a bit of a break from tending to their children.

Another clinic has a little fridge that contains snacks in the waiting room. Patients and their families are welcome to help themselves if they are hungry or thirsty. When the concept of offering snacks was brought up to administration, they responded, "Well, people will abuse this and steal the food." The answer back from the staff was, "If people are hungry or thirsty when they come to our clinic, shouldn't we simply give them food?" The resourceful clinic manager went to the foundation to make a pitch for a budget for snacks and voilà. The clinic now offers sustenance to those who are hungry.

The waiting room process can be softened too. It is like purgatory to sit there and wait for an unknown period of time.

Some clinics have instituted systems that release patients so they can go grab a coffee or go for a walk until the doctor is ready to see them. This can be done simply by handing out restaurant-style pagers that go off when it is time to be seen, or by using electronic tracking methods online, so you can see when your number comes up when it is time for your appointment.

Even restaurants now text your cell phone when they are ready to seat you. Surely the health system could learn from the restaurant industry about improving the waiting experience. At the very least, could there be an indication from the receptionist about how long the wait might be?

I am often cranky, stressed and anxious when I enter a health care setting. I wonder if some of my bad mood could be mitigated by simply being welcomed into a peaceful environment. It strikes me that less cranky patients would help everybody – patient, families and staff too.

First Impressions

∽ the power of staff who set the first impression ⌒

It is only with the heart that one can see rightly.
What is essential is invisible to the eye.
– Antoine de Saint-Exupéry

I watch unit clerks and receptionists carefully. The way in which patients and families are greeted sets the tone for the rest of the experience. I have many stories about botched first impressions.

Aaron was hospitalized when he was six years old to get his tonsils and adenoids removed for sleep apnea. While a T & A (the amusing medical name for a tonsillectomy and adenoidectomy) seems routine, any surgery is a big deal for patients and families. Thinking of my sweet boy suspended in a near-death state when he was under anesthesia is no walk in the park. The children's hospital didn't allow families in the recovery room, so we had to meet him upstairs in the nursing unit at an appointed time.

After his surgery was done, I breathlessly presented at the nursing desk to find out what room he was in. There were a number of people sitting at the desk with their heads down. Nobody looked up at me.

"Excuse me?" I asked tentatively, in close to a tearful state. Finally, a woman reluctantly looked up.

"I'm looking for my son. He just came back from surgery," I squeaked.

"Oh, are you the T & A?" this unknown person of power asked me. Luckily, I had taken a medical terminology course and knew what this meant.

"My son had a T & A, yes."

"Oh," the person of power said dismissively. "He's in room 4D," she said, waving her arm vaguely down the hall.

First impressions. Mean. A lot.

There's one clinic at a children's hospital that had a terrible reputation for rude reception staff. Sure enough, when my son and I presented for an appointment, the receptionist was miserable, saying as little as possible to me, not acknowledging my son at all and waving us towards the equally miserable waiting room. I wondered if the workplace culture there was rotten and this had affected her. Maybe she was going through her own personal problems? I tried to think of reasons for this behaviour. Mostly I thought, "This is your job to care for people. You signed up for this. I did not."

A friend and I met in a downtown coffee shop, swapping stories about health care. This included tales about hospitals using fax machines, notoriously cranky receptionists in clinics, adventures sitting in waiting rooms with small wiggly children for four hours, and the hoops we have to jump through just to get access to our children's own health information. There was really nothing we could do but dissolve into giggles over our lattes.

I recounted a story at a walk-in clinic. I was given a deli counter number by the receptionist at the front desk. This receptionist excelled at using as few words as possible to interact with patients:

Receptionist: "Name?"

Me: "Um, I've never been here before."

Receptionist: "Fill out this form."

Me: Fills out form and brings it back.

Receptionist: (Nothing. Hands me my deli counter number).

I sat for one and a half hours, which maybe isn't that bad? I mostly stared at my deli counter number, which was 70. After the number 69 was called, I looked up in anticipation.

Receptionist (not looking up or standing up or gesturing): "70. Room 4."

I was 70. I was to go to Room 4. I got up and staggered there unaccompanied. I wasn't sure whether to keep the door open or whether to put on a gown or where to sit. The doctor came in, swabbed my throat, and three minutes later, I was in the pharmacy with a prescription clutched in my hand.

This receptionist managed to trim down his number of words used in our interaction to a grand total of eight words. Being called "70" was a new thing for me. Was this approach indicative of the strive towards efficiency? In calling me "70" instead of "Sue Robins," the staff member did save about 0.3 seconds of time. I'd say he saved another 15 seconds by not accompanying me to the treatment room. Ah, but how this efficiency trumped empathy.

I do not know how to even begin to start analyzing this from a patient centred point of view, so I'll just let this sad little tale stand alone.

The Blocks to Really Listening

~ helping patients be stronger when they leave ⌒

I had the chance to really talk with a patient today.
When I say "talk", I mean "listen" and when I say
"a patient", I mean a person.

– Kim Meeking

T he foundation of all health care interactions is built from a patient's and a health care professional's personal values. All humans haul baggage around with them that affects how they interact with other people.

When clinicians say that they have the "best interest of the patients" in mind, I counter – what if the patients have their own best interests in mind instead? Can we help them figure out what that is to them?

A key component is the recognition that as a health professional, you are only a blip in a patient's life. I have made the mistake of saying to health professionals, "This is a job for you, you go home at the end of the day – for patients, this is their life." My error was in my phrasing – passionate professionals tell me that their job is so much more than a job to them. I do not deny this. So I rephrase, "What you do with patients is very important, and I applaud you for making sure your time with them is the best possible quality. Still, patients eventually get discharged away from your care, and then they are on their own."

Why not focus on helping them become stronger in all ways when they walk out your door than when they first came in? This can help them on their greater journey.

My mistake was to minimize the health professional's role and I regret that. Sometimes I put my foot in my mouth too. I do stand by my assertion that clinicians are but blips in a patient's life.

Every year I tell my son's teacher at his school, "This year is really important and you can make a big difference to Aaron's learning and his life." We want to make sure that everything that happens with Aaron this year contributes to our bigger picture – his quest for friendships, a girlfriend, his need for independence and employment. Aaron himself (and his family) are in this for the long haul.

We have had many health professionals make a difference in our lives, like Dr. Darwish, Dr. Lewis, countless nurses and therapists – I regret I cannot remember all their names. They have helped our family be stronger upon leaving than when we first came. What they did in the moment was important, as was the realization that ultimately they leave us too. Offering us tools, like insider knowledge of the system or connections to other patients and families, helps us to continue on after they were long gone.

Every Word Matters

∽ how patients are talked to matters a lot ⌒

Simplicity is the ultimate in sophistication.

– Unknown

C leveland Clinic, known for their leadership in patient centred
care, has released a video about language in health care. In
Words Matter, patients and families give examples of ways that words
from health care professionals have helped them and harmed them.[1]

> *"The way that they told me, it was like they didn't even care. They
> didn't even think about how they were saying it."*

> *"He was in a hurry. He just talked to me for a second and then
> he walked out of the room," says one man describing his cancer
> diagnosis.*

Contrast with these more positive approaches:

> *"She was talking with me, not at me."*

> *"He was real gentle....he hugged me and that put me at ease."*

The video ends with the question: by what words will you be
remembered?

Dr. Naomi Rosenberg published a poignant essay called *How to Tell a Mother Her Child is Dead*. In it, she gives a vivid first-person account about what it is like as a doctor to tell a mother in the emergency department that her child has died. She talks about practicing, recognizing the gravity of the situation, not rushing, sitting down, listening, leaving silence and sharing facts but using careful language.[2]

Rosenberg ends with, "When you leave the room, do not yell at the medical student who has a question. When you get home, do not yell at your husband. If he left his socks on the floor again today, it is all right."

Her essay demonstrates how health care is about relationships between human beings; therefore the interaction must reflect a human approach. The physician's deep respect for the mother and for the child who died is laden in the approach and the words chosen to share the news.

Any anger I might have felt towards my own physician during Aaron's Down syndrome diagnosis disappeared after I read this essay. I finally understood how it felt for clinicians to share news. Having understanding for each other can also foster empathy for each other.

Many people asserted that I was brave and strong after my cancer diagnosis. This was puzzling to me. I was brave to pick up the phone and listen to my doctor tell me my diagnosis? I was strong to follow my various physicians' recommendations about what to do next?

There was nothing in having cancer that made me a hero. The one thing I guess I did was persevere. I plowed through. I didn't give up. I dutifully showed up early to all my appointments. I endured the needles. I changed my dressings. I laid as still as possible under the radiation machine and held my breath for 30 seconds at a time, as I was told.

I did my best to be a good patient. The "brave and strong" words were not helpful to me. They made me feel pressured to be cheerful all the time and they did not allow me any room to express that

I was sad or scared. I was sad and scared. Those words, brave and strong, put me in a box.

Patients meander through the illness experience, often called the journey. I'm not positive that all patients like the language of the journey. The same is true for the fighting metaphors kicking around, particularly in the cancer world.

The whole cancer as a journey language doesn't sit well with me. Neither do the words survivor or warrior or cancer-free. The only phrase that fits with me was person who has breast cancer, but even that phrase is troublesome. A more accurate description would be: person who had breast cancer, but still might have it floating around in her body somewhere but nobody has found it yet. That's quite a mouthful.

It is just best to make no assumptions about what language a person wants to use, because every person is different. Taking the person's lead by listening closely to their own use of language is a good start.

Every word matters in the disability world too.

Disabled people and their families can be particular about language and for good reason. I think it is because it is the one thing in our out-of-control lives that we can control.

Even better than listening to me as a mom, it is best to listen to the disabled person themselves. Aaron says he is Down syndrome, not that he has Down syndrome. He should have the final say in how he is referred to.

Words are powerful. Patients need to have control over how they are named and described. I'm not the breast cancer patient in room five. I'm Sue, a scared, middle-aged mom who has just been diagnosed with breast cancer. Using person-first language can show respect for a patient as a person.

For those who are disabled, it is best to research recommendations about language written by different disability communities. For instance, many autistic people do not like person-first language. I know all this might be confusing. If you aren't sure about what language to use, the best thing to do is to ask.

What do patients want? It depends. Everybody is different. I do know that the words chosen by health professionals are remembered forever. Please choose them carefully.

Notes

1. Cleveland Clinic, Words Matter, https://www.youtube.com/watch?v=SyIuAMzao6M
2. Rosenberg, Naomi, How to Tell a Mother her Child is Dead, September 2016, https://www.nytimes.com/2016/09/04/opinion/sunday/how-to-tell-a-mother-her-child-is-dead.html

Make Space for the Suffering

∽ the importance of not turning away from patient suffering ∽

I like the idea of songs sung by those without big voices.
You know, small birdsongs that rise above the noise of the city.

– *Kyo Maclear*

I 've had stumbles in my ordinary life—a divorce, big moves, lost jobs, and financial woes. When I've fallen, I've always slowly gotten back up. The year I got cancer I was brought to my knees, and I struggled to rise again.

When my doctor called that snowy day in February to tell me I had breast cancer, I fell into a black hole of physical and emotional pain. Cancer starkly reminded me that nobody is guaranteed a pain-free life. Along with my diagnosis and treatment came suffering that was chained to my unexpected state of illness. Previously, I had shunned the word suffering. The phrase "burden and suffering" has been slapped onto the backs of people with disabilities for a very long time. I have strongly asserted that my son is not a burden nor has he been suffering. Society and systems remain his burdens.

My own cancer has forced me to reconsider the notion of suffering. Suffering is such a loaded word. If suffering means experiencing a threat to oneself, we all suffer at some point in our lives. In recounting my recent experiences in health care, I am struck by the many instances of unmitigated suffering that I endured in the hospital. I almost passed out from an unsedated fine wire insertion in my breast. A receptionist sternly scolded me. The nurse wouldn't allow my husband in the room to hold my hand during an IV start. I unexpectedly had a needle full of blue dye injected into my nipple. A young radiation therapist chastised me. At the same time, I was struggling with my identity of suddenly being a sick person and looking my own mortality in the eye. I was often cold, in physical pain, and terribly alone.

Health professionals are taught to be fixers and heroes. My suffering seemed to make many clinicians uncomfortable. I was told, "You have a good kind of cancer." "You are lucky they caught it early." "Be positive." "Be brave." "Be strong." I felt anything but strong: I was weak, vulnerable, and dependent. This is the unspoken nature of cancer and many other illnesses too. My husband and children remind me how families are bound together through thick and thin. When a loved one hurts, the other loved ones hurt, but in their own unique way.

My husband tells me he wouldn't describe his own experience with my illness as suffering, but watching me suffer has caused him to be upset, worried, and uncertain. He describes the time between diagnosis and surgery as terrifying. He settled down during my treatment because he felt I was being looked after. His emotional stress has resurfaced as I grappled post-treatment with my own value and worth. I realize that nobody ever asked my husband about his emotional pain. He came with me to all of my medical appointments. Except for introductions, few clinicians spoke to him directly or asked him how he was doing. He often sat invisibly in the chair in the corner of the clinic room.

I call my daughter, who was then a third-year nursing student, to collect her thoughts on suffering. "Suffering is a harsh word," she muses. "But then I think suffering is part of being human." She is wise beyond her years. "I was really sad when you were diagnosed," she continues during our tearful conversation. "It is painful to see the ones you love suffer." She says what helped her was when she had something to do—even small things, like sitting with me, helping me read my pre-op pamphlets, or changing my dressing after my surgery. She says it is important for family members to feel acknowledged and useful.

The love of my husband and children has taught me that kindness is a salve for emotional suffering. There were small moments of kindness in my cancer experience in health care. The mammogram tech stroked my hair during my biopsy. The radiation therapist covered me with a warm blanket before treatment. My medical oncologist gave me an impromptu hug. My family physician randomly phoned just to see how I was doing.

In contrast, there seemed to be no space to acknowledge my pain within the hospital environment. I felt like I was just another generic breast cancer patient. My breast surgeon had no time to see me after my surgery. I was in and out of my oncologist's office within minutes. My radiation therapy appointments were only 12 minutes long. I was allotted only four counseling appointments with the therapist at the cancer hospital.

I was wholly unprepared for all of this. Not one clinician sat me down to say, "This is hard." My tumour was treated well, but as the person who carried the tumour, I was rarely considered. I thought I was losing my mind. It wasn't until I finally spoke to a therapist that I was told, "All that you are feeling is normal." "Really?" I said tentatively.

"Yes," she said firmly and added, "You are minimizing your own pain. Let's talk about it."

"Let's talk about it." Four small words.

I only began healing from cancer when I was given permission to feel again, to not be strong, and was allowed to acknowledge my own suffering. Avoiding pain does not make it go away. How I wish that I had encountered somebody that sat down, looked me in the eye, took my hand, and said to me, "How are you really feeling? Let's talk about it." That person could have been anyone who works in a health care setting. It should not only be the mental health professionals who are tasked with acknowledging our emotional pain. Healers turn toward patients and families during their pain. A warm gesture, kind word, or gentle touch reminds us that we are not alone and makes space for our suffering. While health care can (sometimes) cure, it is love that will heal us in the end.

A version of this essay was originally published in the Journal of Family Nursing, February 2018.
Robins, Sue, Make Space for Suffering, Journal of Family Nursing (Volume: 24, Issue: 1, pp. 3-7). Copyright ©2018, Sue Robins. DOI: https://doi.org/10.1177/1074840717754300.

There Is No Gold Standard

~ comparing pediatric and adult health care ~

Very great change starts from very small
conversations held among people who care.

– *Margaret Wheatley*

I was surprised to learn that the elements of good care in the
pediatric disability world are the exact same in the adult cancer
world. Fundamental notions like respect, dignity, information sharing and partnership are universal, no matter how old you are. And
why wouldn't they be universal? How do things change the moment
you turn 18 years-old? Sadly, the adult system has not embraced
patient centred care as the pediatric world has. I assumed that adult
cancer treatment would be better.

I learned that cancer care suffers from the same challenges as the
rest of health care. In my experience, there is no gold standard in
cancer care. It is just health care like everywhere else, with struggles
with funding, pressures to be efficient, and handling of big egos. I
received no special care because I had cancer. For the staff treating
cancer patients, it was just another day at work. They had seen thou-

sands of cancer patients and my cancer wasn't even the worst cancer they'd encountered.

Breast cancer is a dime a dozen. The aggressive breast cancer awareness campaigns do not serve breast cancer patients. In fact, the opposite has happened – people say, "Oh breast cancer,"; shrug – that's treatable – whatever, you'll be fine – and that is that. To staff at the cancer hospital, cancer was simply ordinary, a part of their typical day.

Contrast that to how a patient feels after a cancer diagnosis. To start, I was a person who suddenly became a patient. I had no overt symptoms, except for my ridge, and I did not even feel sick. My treatment would make me sick.

Then, cancer forced me to look my own mortality right in the eye. Yes, we are all going to die in some vague, undated future. Cancer slaps you across the face and says, "Guess what, sucker? You are going to die sooner rather than later. Your own body has turned against you in the most sinister of ways. All those things on your bucket list? You should have done them by now." This "You are gonna die" messaging from my cancer made me feel like I had my head in a slowly closing vise.

In this state, with the head in the vise, in hospital settings, I realized that I was very good at speaking up for my son, but I had no idea how to speak up for myself. I was run over like a head-on collision with cancer. In my fragile state, I dropped my advocate veneer and felt very small.

I came to the stark realization that while I had sympathy for my son when he had health care encounters, I had been lacking in empathy. Health care experiences are often traumatic, tests and treatments are brutal, great pain is inflicted without relief, and even the thought of an appointment is very anxiety-provoking. I know that now – I think I didn't realize the depth of pain that health care can inflict, and I now will talk with Aaron about those realities and feelings instead of just bribing him with French fries to go to the lab to get his blood taken.

As I attended more and more appointments, I tried to worry less about being liked. I was less apologetic and more direct.

I learned how to breathe and meditate while waiting for the doctor to come in the treatment room or while lying underneath the radiation machine. I've been forced to learn all sorts of ways to tackle anxiety – breathing, walking, meditating – that I hope I can teach Aaron too. I also re-learned the value of having peers who can laugh with you about the ridiculousness of the health system – other women with breast cancer who can laugh about having blue dye in our nipples for months, or friends with kids in the disability world who can laugh at the ridiculousness of fax machines, appointment cards sent in the mail, and being called by a number, not a name, in a clinic. I need to laugh as well as cry.

This book is my healing. If one health care student or professional reads this, reflects on their own behaviour and adjusts it just a tiny bit to offer more compassion to patients, I will be happy. If one patient or family member reads my words and it inspires them to tell their story about what's important to them, I'll be happy too. If one health administrator is reminded that health care is about human beings, not data, then my job is done. If my husband or kids read this and come away with a strong sense of how much I love them, then I will die a happy woman.

Advocate Me

∽ my struggles to advocate for myself ⌣

**...a magnificent cause can overcome a prickly
personality, but why make things harder?**
– Guy Kawasaki

I never wanted to be an advocate. I'm a conflict-averse introvert by nature. When my youngest son was born with Down syndrome, the title of "advocate" was foisted upon me. I was also suddenly a Special Needs Mom. These were clubs I never signed up for.

Thrown neck-deep into the health system with a baby with medical issues, I quickly learned to speak up at specialists' offices to get my questions answered. I figured out that most advocacy work is relationship-based.

I got to know my son's clinicians and recognized the value of chitchat, being nice, giving thank you cards and remembering people's birthdays.

I've been to protests and marches to call for fair government funding for people with disabilities. I've spoken to the media about policies that segregate my kid. I lobbied a children's hospital to start up a medical Down syndrome clinic and then fought hard when an administrator tried to shut it down a few years later. I have a fierce reputation as a strong advocate and I would take a bullet for any of my children.

Yet my advocacy efforts came to a screeching halt when I was diagnosed with breast cancer. Many friends said, "Watch out, cancer world, strong advocate Sue Robins is here" – but that bravado did not come to pass. I've often failed miserably at advocating for myself as a cancer patient.

It had been easier to advocate for my son. He was one step removed from me, and I could hide behind my role of the strong mama bear. Cancer is exceedingly personal and not one step removed at all, for my own cells have turned rogue on me. Breast cancer is an especially intimate sort of cancer – my breast tumour was an affront to my feminine body.

Sitting in exam rooms in thin gowns, exposing my breasts to strange hands and painful machines, I couldn't figure out a way to salvage my dignity, never mind advocate for myself.

People told me to buck up, to advocate for myself as I had for my son. This call to action was not what I needed; it only served to pile on guilt at my own helplessness. I simply craved compassion instead.

I poked my head back into published writing. A leader in radiation therapy asked me to co-author a journal article about my experience having radiation. A nursing professor asked me to write a guest editorial for her journal about suffering. I am hopeful my story leaves remnants for clinicians to pause and consider how patients feel when they are in their care. While this might not help me, this may help others behind me in the cancer world. Making meaning from my experience helps me heal too.

There are many ways to speak up for ourselves. Some people fundraise, lobby governments, give direct feedback to clinicians or bring along support people to appointments to help them be heard. Other folks just hang in there, endure and try to forget about the whole damn thing. That's okay too.

Just as there's not one right way to do cancer, there's not one right way to advocate. The most important thing is to be kind and forgiving of yourself as you find your own way.

An edited version of this essay was originally published on the Cancer Knowledge Network, February 12, 2018. https://cancerkn.com/advocate-me/

Invincible Summer

~ seeking out care after cancer treatment was done ~

In the midst of winter, I found there was,
within me, an invincible summer.

– Albert Camus

After my cancer treatment, my physical scars began to heal, my hematoma shrunk and my burned skin faded. My mind was not so easily healed.

"Where do I go now?" I sobbed at my last publicly funded appointment. Four sessions were not nearly enough now that cancer had opened my Pandora's box.

"We can't recommend other therapists," I was told. So I turned to Google.

Thankfully, Callanish Society showed up in my search results. I embarked on counselling appointments with my new therapist Susie, trekking across the city for regular sessions as the rest of me slowly began to heal.

I embraced everything about the Callanish house – the streaming light in the building, the warm greeting when I walked in the door, the peaceful hushed atmosphere, the tea offered to me at the start of each session. It was everything I was missing in my patient experience at the hospital.

I signed up for their retreat, but was terrified of the idea of being part of a group. I'm fine in one-on-one situations, but I struggle in larger settings.

The retreat date crept closer. But because of my work in therapy, where my therapist gently guided me through my pain, I was feeling stronger and more resilient. I didn't know what to expect, but I felt ready to be with other people who had cancer too.

To prepare me for the retreat, Susie sagely recommended, "You will have to allow people to be nice to you." As a caregiver, mom to a kid with a disability and a classic nurturer and pleaser – as silly as it sounds – allowing people to be nice to me was a challenge.

Driving up to the gravel parking lot at the retreat location, there was a group of lovely women standing there, smiling and waving, awaiting my arrival. My room was beautifully appointed and tucked away on the second floor of a wooden cottage. There was a massive vase of gorgeous flowers to welcome me. This was my first glimpse into what was to come in the next five days.

We began each day meditating, learning qigong and slowly waking up to the sounds of beautiful crystal singing bowls. There was hard personal group work in the mornings, carefully facilitated by professionals, focused on loss and death. The afternoons were for rest and relaxation – with therapeutic touch, music and counselling. The day was studded with joyful meals, prepared with love by the volunteers in the kitchen. There was camaraderie, laughter and tears. Each day ended with an evening council, where everybody – staff, volunteers and participants – gathered in the great room around the crackling fire.

I was treated with unconditional kindness. I did allow people to be nice to me because I never once felt judged. Just being me seemed enough. It gave me comfort to know that every person working at the retreat was there to share their gifts with us. There was a clear belief in the concept of benevolent service – an approach that is sadly missing in today's health care world. Us retreat participants were not a burden – instead, we felt like a joy. I had a sense that every touch at the retreat was carefully planned and tweaked based on years of wisdom. I wasn't scared because I was safe.

There are fond memories of what remains after the Callanish retreat: I have access to a new serenity inside of me. I don't wake up feeling panicked anymore. When worry crosses my mind (and negative thoughts do still come), I now have tools to pull up to let them wash over me. I can close my eyes and breathe, listen to music, walk in nature, or simply remember my time at the retreat. If I start ruminating on the past or fretting about the future, I pause and centre in the moment. I look up in the sky and think, "It's a beautiful day."

After the retreat, my husband said that I smiled easier. For anxious, tormented me, these newfound skills are the ultimate gift for me and my family. Despite cancer (or maybe because of it?), I have finally found a sliver of peace in my heart.

I understand that hospitals are not going to start offering retreats for cancer patients, at least not here in Canada. I do wonder if there are little elements from a place like Callanish that can be offered in cancer hospitals, like the healing environment, the attention to mental health, the careful nurturing of safe spaces. These tweaks could transform cancer medical treatment into true cancer care.

A version of this essay was originally published in the Callanish Newsletter, June 2018.

All the
Warm Blankets

∾ examples of simple kindnesses that make a big difference ∾

And did you get what
you wanted from this life, even so?
I did.
And what did you want?
To call myself beloved, to feel myself
beloved on the earth.

– Raymond Carver

I remember every single act of kindness I've encountered in health settings over the past years. The images are embedded in my head like bright glowing lights. I revisit them often to comfort me in times of distress and to rekindle hope in health care when my hope begins to wane.

At 4 a.m., when I am dozing in the chair beside my son in the emergency room, I am grateful for the nurse who covered me up with a warm blanket. The warm blankets are my symbol for kindnesses in health care and they mean the world to me.

There are so many ways to share simple acts of kindness, even in

the public spaces in hospitals. I can think of the senior administrator who always lets patients and families in and out of the elevators
first; the nurse who lets patients or families bump in line in front of
her in the coffee lineup; people who make eye contact and smile at
patients in the hallway, comment on cute babies in elevators, and
hold doors open for strollers and wheelchairs; any staff member
or student who take the time to help a lost patient or family. Even
better, the staff who escort lost folks directly to their destination in
the hospital.

If every staff member and student committed to doing one simple
act of kindness every single day for a patient or family member
in the hospital corridors and lobbies, imagine what kind of environment would be created in what is often a rushed, stressful and
confusing place.

Really, anybody working in a health care setting – parking lot
attendants, cafeteria cashiers, receptionists, clinicians – has these
choices to make in every encounter with a patient, a dozen times a
day: do they respond neutrally because they are hiding behind professionalism? Do they respond with cruelness to assert their power
over the vulnerable patient? Or they do respond as a healer, with
demonstrated compassion for those people they signed up to serve?
Demonstrated compassion translates into acts of kindness.

One day, the occupational therapist who supported Aaron when
he was a toddler looked me in the eye and unexpectedly said, "You
are doing a great job as Aaron's mom." I responded to her sentiment
by bursting into grateful tears.

Then there was the OR nurse who ushered me out the door after
Aaron was anesthetized for surgery. She put her hand on my shoulder
and said, "Don't worry, we will take very good care of him for you."

A mammogram technologist stroked my arm when I was administered the sharp freezing for my breast biopsy. Later, she tenderly

brushed my hair when it fell into my face, causing instant tears to well up in my eyes and slowly drip onto the green hospital pillow.

Our family doctor once called me out of the blue just to see how Aaron was doing when he was going through a rough spell. This seems like a little thing, but it was a big thing to me.

When Aaron was hospitalized with pneumonia, he was lucky enough to have an exceptional student nurse assigned to his care. She joked with him, high-fived him and patiently sat with him on his bed while he took his inhaler meds. I later took the time to write a thank you note to her and send a copy to her instructor. Even if the system doesn't reward kindnesses, it doesn't mean that we can't recognize and acknowledge tender care.

During Aaron's hospital stay, the pediatric resident wrote his name on the white board in the room so we wouldn't feel foolish if we forgot his name. A child life volunteer took the time to gown up to come in Aaron's isolation room to fix his video console. An aide stayed with my sleeping boy early one morning so I could run down to get a desperately needed cup of coffee. The nurse on the night shift tiptoed about with a flashlight, minimizing disturbances while making rounds.

None of this is counted by the hospital funders, but all of it matters to me.

A kind manner often does not take more time and it is also free. This is my call to the return of the old-fashioned notion of bedside manner.

The simple stuff matters, every single time. Kindness is not about being nice. It is the demonstration of compassion that is at the core of patient and family centred care.

We all are softened by compassion. It rubs out the hard edges in this messed-up beautiful world. Give us your kindnesses, in any form they take. They are salve for my wounds, if only for a moment.

As Evidenced by His Smile

∾ how a smiling lab tech turned my experience upside-down ∽

What you don't know you can feel it somehow.

– U2

I had a rotten follow-up appointment at the oncology clinic. The oncologist seemed annoyed with me from the moment she walked in the door. I did not know whether she was having a bad day or if it was me that was annoying her with all my stupid questions. I left the oncology clinic worn down. I shuffled across the street to the cancer hospital to get my blood drawn, just wanting the whole afternoon to be over. This was a day to be endured. I hate being a patient.

I sat in the waiting room and the lab tech came out and called my name. I had my head down and was feeling small and dejected. I looked up and he was smiling at me. In my current state, this made me nervous. I smiled back, just a little bit. He smiled wider. This smiling business was contagious. Here was someone who seemed actually happy to see me. I didn't feel like an intrusion or bother to him as evidenced by his smile. I could feel myself start to relax.

He walked me to the lab and invited me to sit down. "What arm would you like?" "Um, right," I said, "I'm left-handed." (I don't know what difference that makes, but I was feeling a wee bit less guarded and thought I'd dip my toe into some conversation). "I'm left-handed too!" he said, delighted. We concluded that means we are both creative. We smiled at each other some more.

I didn't even feel the needle go into my arm. He praised my veins and asked about my Christmas. "How many kids do you have?" he asked. And later, "I can't believe you have a 25-year-old!" I was still smiling, feeling a bit silly that I was so easily flattered. My mood was shifting. I was now feeling considerably better, sitting in a chair at the cancer hospital getting poked by a needle for five vials of blood.

This kindness was such a contrast from my appointment across the street with the oncologist. This young lab tech went to school for two years to be a medical laboratory technician. The Internet tells me he probably makes less than $30 an hour. He's near the bottom of the hospital pecking order. My oncologist went to school for more than ten years and is one of the queens of the hill at the hospital, status-wise. She makes considerably more than $30 an hour. Guess which experience with which person I'd rather spend my time thinking and writing about?

This lab tech has much to teach the rest of the health care world about connecting with and caring for patients. I feel deeply grateful for him.

To health professionals everywhere, know this: your compassion is evidenced by your smile.

Be Kinder
Than You Think
is Necessary

∽ my hope placed in the new generation of clinicians ⌒

Be kinder to yourself.
And then let your kindness flood the world.

– Pema Chödrön

I presented once to second-year medical students. At the end of my talk, one student asked, "What is the one thing you want us to remember?' I paused, fearing I had shared about fifty things too many with them – they only wanted the one take-away, the one thing that they might be tested on.

I thought for a moment, nervous about distilling an hour-long presentation into one sentence. "Be kinder than you think is necessary," I said. This was the saying engraved on a little plaque that sits on my windowsill. If these students could do one thing when they were working with patients, I hoped that it was to be kind.

This is the hard part of health care. Health care is so task-based that the acts of kindness are not properly acknowledged or counted by funders or administrators. Workload measurement systems collect a health professional's tasks: taking vital signs, charting, collecting a history. There's no workload measurement for holding an old lady's hand or giving someone a hug. The health care system doesn't value these activities. But patients and families do.

"What do you do in the hospital?" I ask my daughter Ella when she was in the first year of her nursing education.

"Well, today I sat with an older lady who was a patient there," she replied. "She was hard of hearing, but she loved to talk. So I sat and listened to her." Later in her placement, she told me shyly "The lady I was assigned to gave me a hug." I felt tears well in my eyes and my heart grew three times its regular size. My daughter is becoming the kind of nurse who I want to see when I go to the hospital. This is what a good nurse looks like to me.

Instead of expecting their students to run through a litany of tasks during this first placement, Ella's university chose to give opportunities for students in their first clinical placements to sit with their assigned patients and simply talk to them. I love this philosophy. It is the person who matters first, not the blood pressure. The blood pressure can come later.

By arranging a curriculum to value the people first by teaching the tasks later, this nursing faculty sets the tone for these impressionable students about what's most important in health care. And that's the people. I have an inkling that true change in health care will come first by looking at the types of students recruited to health faculties. Then it will come with allowing them opportunities early in their education to experience the care part of health care, which means scheduling the time to sit by a patient's bedside, simply listening to them talk.

Love is the Answer

∿ how love fits into health care ᔐ

This is not wasted time. It is the work we do.

– Kirsten Meisinger

Twenty-eight years after my post-grad studies in health care administration, 17 years after my work experience at the ministry of health, 16 years after the birth of my youngest son with an extra chromosome, 14 years after my work as a volunteer on a family council, 11 years after the start of my family engagement career, two years after my breast cancer diagnosis, I have finally found the answer I have been looking for.

What is the key to partnering with people, patient and family centred care, patient engagement, patient experience, patient satisfaction and communication? Love. Love is the answer, my friends.

Five years ago, I read a profound essay called *Love: A word that medicine fears*, written by a family physician named Kirsten Meisinger. Dr. Meisinger finally uttered the word that I'd been skirting around all these years. I had been speaking about listening, holding space, perspective taking, empathy, caring, compassion, and humanity in health care. These are all euphemisms for one word: love.[1]

"Funny thing is, once you start openly loving patients – once you

open yourself – you become more effective, not less," Dr, Meisinger emphasizes. "This is not wasted time. It is the work we do. We
change people, make them care more for themselves and their
health by openly caring for them first."

I will care for myself if I myself feel cared for.

Love means a deep caring for patients, their families, each other
and ourselves. If we can open our hearts to those who are fragile,
vulnerable and in pain, we will change the landscape of the health
care world. This means dismantling the brick walls around our
hearts that are built by egos, perfectionism, professionalism and
fear. This means demonstrating what is in your heart by a gentle
touch, a kind word, or a thoughtful gesture.

Love is the great revolution in health care, for love is what is at the
very core of health care.

Here's what health professionals can do: create space, time, systems and environments where caring is celebrated, encouraged and
rewarded. Model the compassionate culture you want to see by being compassionate to people lost in the hallways, the housekeeping
staff, your colleagues and yourself. Make the time to actively listen
to people's stories. Don't wait for the system to do this for you. This
is a personal action – you must step up yourself.

Managers, offer to staff the time to be still, reflect and acknowledge their own suffering so they can be open to another's pain.
Teach our students well to lend their young hearts to those in need,
and how to softly save love for themselves so they can go home to
their families at night. Count empathies, not efficiencies. Shed
artificial roles to make person-to-person connections, not provider
to patient ones.

All this love will build and build, until it finally reaches the tip-
ping point. Only then will we get to the true purpose of health care,
and that is to care for other human beings. The answer to all of your

struggles lives in your own hearts. If you slow down, close your eyes and be still, you will hear it whispering to you.

To those who say: health care is much more complicated than that, I say, no, no it is not. Health care is first about human relationships between those who suffer and those who have committed to care. This transcends bureaucrats and budgets, for love is absolutely free.

Love is what heals people. Medicine can sometimes cure. But it cannot heal. It is the gentle hearts that will create change in this beautiful, messed-up world.

Notes
1. Meisinger, Kirsten, Love: A word that medicine fears, November 2012, https://www.kevin-md.com/blog/2012/11/love-word-medicine-fears.html.

The Dude

∿ my kid with Down syndrome grows up ↶

I love you to the universe and back.

–Aaron

When I had cancer, Aaron stepped up to care for me. I hope it wasn't too traumatic for him. With him, you never know. He's not forthright with his feelings. The dude talks, but only reluctantly.

At the beginning of the cancer ordeal, he woke up every morning and asked me, "How is your boob doing today?" How mortifying for a teenage boy to bear witness to everybody talking about his mom's breast. The idea of cancer cells was very confusing to explain to him. He loves science so we told him I had a bad virus. He gave me more hugs, carried the groceries, said he loves me and danced with me in the kitchen more than he ever did before.

One day I confessed to him, "I'm feeling yucky." He responded, "You are not yucky. You are beautiful." Aaron, the one always cared for by others, has learned to be a caregiver too.

Aaron is now 16 years old. He's got the teenage swagger. He's sometimes sullen and often mortified by his mother, whether she had cancer or not. This is all the schtick of regular adolescence. The extra chromosome that comes with Down syndrome hasn't affected this one bit.

I am ashamed to admit that when Aaron was first diagnosed, I began my job being his mom in deep grief about having a disabled kid. This is wholly due to my own ableism, my own stereotypes about people with disabilities. Interestingly, my husband rolled casually with Aaron's diagnosis. One of my husband's old girlfriends had a sister with Down syndrome, so he saw Aaron as a human being, just like everyone else. I struggled mightily with Aaron's diagnosis for years, mostly treading water to keep on top of my own ignorance.

When Aaron was a wee sprog, he was full of energy. He beetled around everywhere, escaping from the house, digging cat litter into his dump truck, finding mischief wherever he went. He had sleep apnea for the first six years of his life, barely slept and required constant supervision. I was one tired mother.

Slowly, slowly, as he got older, he settled down and matured. I think it took him a few years to get used to Planet Earth, which is often hostile to people with disabilities. If I'm honest, it took us all a while to get used to each other.

The recent teenage years have been challenging but wonderful. Everybody grows up. Why was it a shock when Aaron hit puberty? Had I thought he would remain a child forever? (I think so). It has been a joy to watch him blossom into a fledgling adult. He has become more himself, which is funny, quick with words, a snappy dresser and an emotionally-astute people person. He is a joy to be around.

Aaron will proudly tell you that he is an actor. He has been signed by a talent agent and has been auditioning for roles on film and television. He recently shot his first commercial. We are waiting for the entertainment business to catch up to the concept of diversity with disabled people. We know it is coming.

In the meantime, he is working on his craft. The improvisation community has welcomed him with open arms and he has regular sessions with an acting coach who believes in him. He goes to casting calls, chewing on his nails in the waiting room like all the other actors. He marches into the auditions alone and always ends up making the casting directors laugh.

I have moved through various stages of being the mother of a child with Down syndrome: from tolerance to acceptance and finally to celebration. We no longer care if people stare at Aaron in the mall. (And yes, they still do stare). We've taught him to stare right back. He's a confident young man. He says that acting makes him feel alive. We will put our eggs in that basket and will take it as far as it goes.

As Natalie Merchant says in her song Wonder, with love, patience and faith, he will make his own way. Our children make their own way whether they have 46 chromosomes or 47. Aaron is his own man. And he's going to be more than okay.

My Shining Glimmer of Hope

~ my deep admiration for the new generation ~

**Sometimes the world is so beautiful I have
to shoot rainbows out of my eyes.**

– Russell Alton

My daughter Ella graduated from her Bachelor of Science in Nursing program in June. At her ceremony, I sat in the balcony of the hall with Aaron. We dressed in our finest, bursting with pride, looking out over the sea of black convocation hats below us. This class of nursing graduates signified an infusion of hope for the health care world.

This is a new generation of smart, compassionate nurses. Ella has been called to serve for patients and their families. She did not choose an easy career. At her tender age, she already has borne close witness to untold suffering. She has given injections, changed dressings, started IVs and wrapped up bodies of the deceased. In her career, she will welcome babies and hold vigil during people's last breaths.

My wish for my daughter is that she remains open-hearted while being kind and true to herself.

Ella is quiet and soft-spoken. She has always been an old soul, wise beyond her years. She is a great observer of people and has mastered the fine art of listening. I know that nursing was hard work for her, physically, intellectually and emotionally. Her degree is a tremendous accomplishment. Nursing is the toughest undergraduate degree there is.

If you ask Ella why she chose nursing, she says simply, "It is because of Aaron." That is all. That is enough.

A few short weeks after her graduation, Ella was hired as a registered nurse at a children's hospital. She is now working 12-hour shifts and caring for children and families in their worst moments. I am proud of her for achieving her goal of becoming a pediatric nurse. She achieved what I could not. She is a full nurse and I will forever remain half of one.

Witnessing Ella and her classmates walk across that stage to receive their degrees allowed me to settle down and take a deep breath. For the first time in all my years as a health care advocate, first as a mom and then a cancer patient, I can finally take a rest from trying to change the world. I know that I am in good hands now.

It will be this fresh generation of health professionals with gentle hearts like Ella's that will nudge health care into a softer place – one lovely kindness at a time.

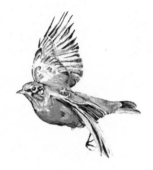

Acknowledgements

Love the ones you are with.

I t was a lonely process to write these stories but it sure took a village to create this book.

I am indebted to Dr. Catherine Crock for her encouragement over the years to get this damn book out of my head and onto paper. Michelle Phillips was my editor who did the heavy lifting to structurally edit this book and Ben Phillips provided valuable publishing advice.

Aaron Mumby generously crafted this design and Bobbie Mumby was the book's layout wizard. The lovely bird illustrations are from talented East Vancouver artist Jacqueline Robins. Tara Hogue Harris used her mad editing skills to copy edit the book. Aaron Loehrlein and Jodine Perkins worked their Library Science magic. Ryan Walter Wagner's photos captured my good side.

I want to express my heartfelt appreciation to many folks.

Laurene Black, Dawn Wrightson and Heather Mattson McCrady gave me my start in family centred care consulting. Lisa Hawthornthwaite and Kate Robson have supported my career along the way.

My dear mom friends, Helga Woywitka, Isabel Jordan, Carmen Welta, Melissa Steele, Karen Calhoun and Jill Howey have accompanied me on my walks in the forest, whether in person or on the phone.

My peers in the patient and caregiving world have informed this work: Lelainia Lloyd, Kimberly Strain, Karen Copeland, Jennifer

Baumbusch, Mary Morgan, Katherine Pratt and Laura White.

Thank you to Susie Merz and Deanna Vernelli for listening to me during my darkest hours.

I want to acknowledge my family. Aaron, my teenage son, for showing me the way to joy. Ella, my only girl, for giving me hope through her dedication and commitment as a pediatric nurse. May she keep her gentle heart intact. Isaac, my eldest son, for sharing his musician's wisdom: Mom, just keep doing your best work. The rest will fall into place.

Extra props to Ella's husband Eisech and Isaac's wife Vicky for encouraging their mother-in-law. My sister from another mother Jacqui and her husband Randy have shown me steadfast support as my extended family.

Finally, I am deeply grateful to my husband Mike for his unwavering enthusiasm for all of my writing. He loves me unconditionally just the way I am. With him I feel invincible. This book would never would have come to life without you my love.

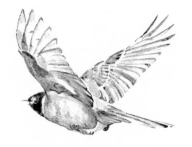

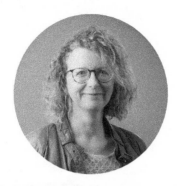

About the Author

Author Sue Robins' career began as a young hospital volunteer and student nurse before she embarked on a series of health administration roles. She was unexpectedly immersed in health care as a caregiver when her third child was born with Down syndrome. In 2017, Sue became a patient when she was diagnosed with breast cancer.

Sue's writing has been widely published, including in *The New York Times*, *The Globe and Mail*, the *Canadian Medical Association Journal*, the *Journal of Family Nursing*, the *Journal of Paediatric and Child Health* and the *Journal of Medical Imaging and Radiation Sciences*. She has spoken at many national and international health conferences about patient and family centred care.

Her recent work experience includes paid family leadership positions with the B.C. Children's Hospital and the Stollery Children's Hospital. Sue is also a senior partner with Bird Communications, a Canadian health communications company.

Sue uses the pronouns she/her and is the mom of three children – Isaac, Ella and Aaron. She lives with her husband and youngest son just outside of Vancouver, Canada on the unceded territory of the Traditional Coast Salish Lands, including the Tsleil-Waututh, Kwikwetlem, Squamish and Musqueam Nations.

CPSIA information can be obtained
at www.ICGtesting.com
Printed in the USA
LVHW030011071119
636609LV00001B/5